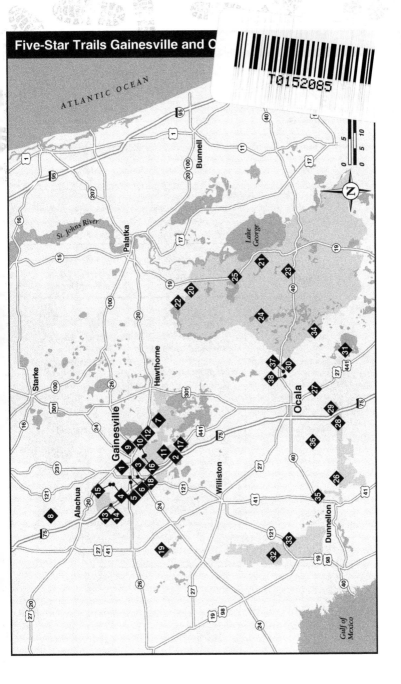

Five-Star Trails Gainesville and O...

T0152085

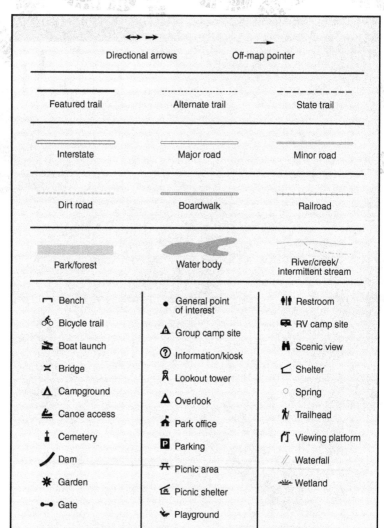

Directional arrows   Off-map pointer

Featured trail   Alternate trail   State trail

Interstate   Major road   Minor road

Dirt road   Boardwalk   Railroad

Park/forest   Water body   River/creek/
intermittent stream

⊓ Bench
⚙ Bicycle trail
🛥 Boat launch
⋈ Bridge
▲ Campground
🛶 Canoe access
⚱ Cemetery
╱ Dam
✳ Garden
●–● Gate

● General point
of interest
⚠ Group camp site
? Information/kiosk
🗼 Lookout tower
▲ Overlook
🏠 Park office
P Parking
🎋 Picnic area
🏠 Picnic shelter
🤸 Playground

♦♦ Restroom
🚐 RV camp site
M Scenic view
⊏ Shelter
○ Spring
🏃 Trailhead
🏛 Viewing platform
// Waterfall
🌿 Wetland

Overview Map Key

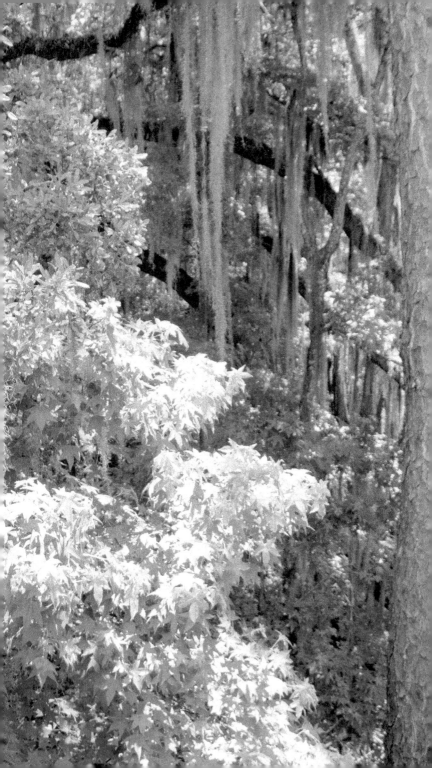

Five-Star Trails

Gainesville & Ocala

Your Guide to the Area's Most Beautiful Hikes

Sandra Friend
and John Keatley

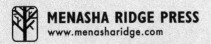

MENASHA RIDGE PRESS
www.menasharidge.com

Five-Star Trails Gainesville & Ocala
Your Guide to the Area's Most Beautiful Hikes

Copyright © 2014 by Sandra Friend
All rights reserved
Published by Menasha Ridge Press
Distributed by Publishers Group West
Printed in the United States of America
First edition, first printing

Cover design and cartography: Scott McGrew
Text design: Annie Long
Cover photograph: Sandra Friend
Interior photographs: Sandra Friend and John Keatley
Author photograph: Janet Hensley
Indexer: Rich Carlson

Frontispiece: Wacahoota Forest *(See Hike 11, Paynes Prairie Preserve State Park: Wacahoota Trail, page 87.)*

Library of Congress Cataloging-in-Publication Data
Friend, Sandra.
  Five-star trails : Gainesville & Ocala : your guide to the area's most beautiful hikes / Sandra Friend, John Keatley. — First edition.
      pages cm. — (Five-star trails)
  ISBN 9780897326148 (pbk.); ISBN 9780897326155 (ebook);
  ISBN 9781634042703 (hardcover)
  1. Hiking—Florida—Gainesville Region—Guidebooks. 2. Hiking—Florida—
Ocala Region—Guidebooks. 3. Trails—Florida—Gainesville Region—Guidebooks.
4. Trails—Florida—Ocala Region—Guidebooks. 5. Gainesville Region (Fla.)—
Guidebooks. 6. Ocala Region (Fla.)—Guidebooks. I. Title.
  GV199.42.F62G354 2013
  796.5109759'79—dc23
                                    2013041713

Menasha Ridge Press
An imprint of AdventureKEEN
2204 First Avenue South, Suite 102
Birmingham, AL 35233
menasharidgepress.com

DISCLAIMER
This book is meant only as a guide to select trails in the Gainesville and Ocala area. This book does not guarantee hiker safety in any way—you hike at your own risk. Neither Menasha Ridge Press nor Sandra Friend nor John Keatley is liable for property loss or damage, personal injury, or death that result in any way from accessing or hiking the trails described in the following pages. Please be especially cautious when walking in potentially hazardous terrains with, for example, steep inclines or drop-offs. Do not attempt to explore terrain that may be beyond your abilities. Please read carefully the introduction to this book as well as further safety information from other sources. Familiarize yourself with current weather reports and maps of the area you plan to visit (in addition to the maps provided in this guidebook). Be cognizant of park regulations and always follow them. Do not take chances.

Contents

Ocala National Forest   139

Cross Florida Greenway   179

Ocala & Vicinity   209

Appendixes   255

Dedication

Honoring Kenneth Smith, whose vision and hard work for more than a decade led to a completed 30-mile segment of the Florida Trail spanning the Cross Florida Greenway, which will delight future hikers for generations to come.

Acknowledgments

Working as a team, we were able to tackle most of the trails for this book on our own, but we still had friends cheering us on and coming out to hike with us. Thanks to Ruth Lawler, Linda Taylor, and Marjorie Byron for walking the Florida Trail with us, and to Brickman Way, Bob Jones, and Brack Barker for their suggestions of "best hikes" in their own backyards. Our heartfelt appreciation goes to Joan and Philip Woods for allowing us to use their home as a base camp for several weeks while we juggled a family emergency with mornings spent hiking for this book. We appreciate the hospitality of Dennis Knight and Ruth and John Lawler for quiet stays in their respective cabins in the Ocala National Forest. Thanks, too, to Anna Mikell and Visit Gainesville for making us feel at home in Gainesville, finding us comfortable accommodations at the Sweetwater Branch Inn and the Best Western Gateway Grand when we weren't camping on our own in the area. Our appreciation also goes out to Rick Ehle, David MacManus, and other members of the Florida Botany Facebook group for assisting with and confirming plant identifications. Thanks also to Greg Wiley of Marion County Parks and Recreation, Katharine Forbes at City of Gainesville Parks and Recreation, and Nels Parson at St. Johns Water Management District for their help. Finally, a tip of our hats to the many volunteers involved with Citizen Support Organizations, local volunteer programs, and the Florida Trail Association for keeping these trails open.

Preface

In the late 1960s, two young lives crossed paths in this region of bubbling springs and rolling hills. Sandra's family visited every year, walking for hours around Silver Springs and Rainbow Springs—before the days of theme parks, when they were nature-based attractions with boat rides and native animals—and visiting other natural features such as Paynes Prairie and Juniper Springs. Meanwhile, John had a 50-miler patch to earn as a Boy Scout, so he and the other members of his troop joined the Florida Trail Association and took a long backpacking trip across the Ocala National Forest. This immersion in natural Florida as youngsters stayed with us for a lifetime, shaping our interest in exploring the outdoors. We ran in different circles for decades but crossed paths at Florida Trail Association events, finally getting to know each other at the Big O Hike, the state's longest-running group hike. Out of this friendship came a lot of hiking, finishing up *Five Star Trails: Orlando* together so we could head up to the Appalachian Trail to embark on fulfilling our respective lifelong dreams of an AT thru-hike. While we didn't make it all the way, three months on the trail solidified our partnership—and our relationship.

Sandra's family moved to Ocala in the 1970s, and since then, when she wasn't living in the Orlando metro area or the mountains of western Pennsylvania, she's lived, worked, and hiked around Gainesville and Ocala. In the late 1990s, she worked with Kenneth Smith and Bob Jones building a new 30-mile section of the Florida Trail through Ocala on the Cross Florida Greenway and was honored to represent the hiking community by being among those cutting the green ribbon in 2001 to open the Land Bridge over I-75. For several years, she oversaw trail maintenance of the Pruitt section of the Florida Trail (Hike 26), near her home.

With this deep background in local hiking to draw from, we had a lot of fun with research. While some of Sandra's old favorites didn't make it into the book because the trails just weren't five-star material anymore, we discovered new, amazing landscapes to share, like the vast prairies of Watermelon Pond (Hike 19), the rugged slopes and big trees of Creek Sink (Hike 13), and the massive wetlands at Barr Hammock (Hike 2). Between the richness of the Ocala National Forest, the easy-to-reach hikes along the Cross Florida Greenway, and the wealth of new natural lands conserved around Gainesville over the past decade, we had more than enough places to explore.

Only 35 miles apart as I-75 flies, Gainesville and Ocala share many aspects of natural features and habitats formed from the mix of bedrock and soil throughout the region. Among these are karst features—karst being limestone eroded over time by slightly acidic rainfall—including sinkholes of all shapes and sizes, irregular limestone boulders and rocky bluffs, caverns, creeks that vanish into the earth, and springs. Hikes in this guide showcase many of the most spectacular karst features in the area, including the vast plain of Paynes Prairie. To the north of the prairie, Gainesville sits atop the southern edge of the ancient Northern Highlands of Florida, while to its south, the Central Highlands begin. You'll often hear locals refer to the region as North Central Florida, although it's firmly to the northern part of the Florida peninsula. Atop the highlands are vast rolling hills that, in a few well-protected areas, are still topped with the longleaf pine and wiregrass savannas on which botanist William Bartram commented during his 1774 exploration of the region, as well as diminutive, desertlike scrub forests growing atop ancient sand dunes. Some of the northernmost hikes in this book feel positively Appalachian, with rugged landscapes and the same trees and wildflowers you'd find in North Carolina; other hikes, such as the popular boardwalk between Juniper Springs and Fern Hammock Springs, or the walk through Marshall Swamp, are downright tropical in nature. It's a fascinating region, botanically and visually.

This book is designed for hikers of all abilities. Included are some of the roughest, longest day hikes in this sometimes hilly region, as well as hikes of moderate length and very short strolls that

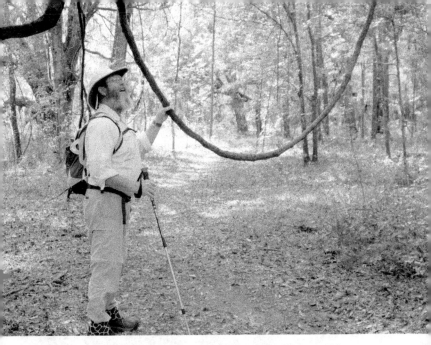

JOHN ADMIRES THE GIANT GRAPEVINES AT SANTOS; *see Hike 27, page 186*

are perfect for families with small children or people with limited mobility. At some parks, you can reward the kids with time on the playground after a short but beautiful walk in the woods. In the wilder places, primitive camping is available along some of the trails, enabling you to turn a day hike into a backpacking experience. All of the hikes can be done in a day, with this caveat: Hikes 26, Florida Trail: Pruitt (pages 180–185), and 22, Florida Trail: Rodman to Lake Delancy (pages 153–159), are best planned as a shuttle so as not to be a prohibitively long day trip; or you can follow the Route Details for advice on where to turn around and retrace your steps to the starting point if you do not have a shuttle car or pickup arrangement.

Always remain aware of the available, seasonal natural light for these day hikes. Be especially mindful when hiking in deeply wooded areas, where darkness prevails earlier than on exposed trails. For example, in late November, if you're headed out on a four-hour hike, don't start walking at 2 p.m.

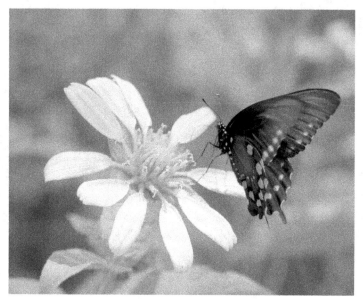

BUTTERFLY AT SILVER SPRINGS STATE PARK; *see Hike 38, page 249*

Known to hikers for its 70-mile segment of the statewide Florida Trail, the Ocala National Forest is the top destination in Florida for backpackers and day hikers. The region's springs have always attracted visitors, with Silver Springs being one of the world's largest (it has been a tourist attraction since the 1860s and is now a state park). Within its city limits, Gainesville has dozens of parks and gentle trails, where residents and visitors alike can take refuge in nature. We've done a lot of exploring to point you to the best of these natural getaways, some of which hide in plain sight. We know that if you enjoy the outdoors, you probably enjoy more than one activity, so we've included sites where, in addition to the hike, you may be able to camp, swim, paddle, or cycle, too. Just as we do on our popular website, **floridahikes.com,** we want to inform, inspire, and nudge you out the door to enjoy Florida's natural areas, so you'll fall in love with our unique blend of ecosystems and want to protect them for future generations.

Recommended Hikes

Best Hikes for Birding

6   Loblolly Woods Nature Park (p. 56)

7   Longleaf Flatwoods Reserve (p. 62)

8   Mill Creek Preserve (p. 68)

30   Marshall Swamp Trail (p. 202)

33   Goethe State Forest: Buck Island Pond Trail (p. 220)

Best Hikes for Botanical Beauty

1   Alfred A. Ring Park (p. 30)

12   Prairie Creek Preserve (p. 92)

13   San Felasco Hammock Preserve State Park:
Moonshine Creek Trails (p. 99)

17   Tuscawilla Preserve (p. 122)

32   Goethe State Forest: Big Cypress Trail (p. 215)

Best Hikes for Dogs

5   John Mahon Nature Park (p. 52)

16   Sweetwater Preserve (p. 117)

27   Florida Trail: Santos (p. 186)

28   Florida Trail: Southwest 49th Avenue to Land Bridge (p. 191)

29   Land Bridge Loop (p. 197)

35   Rainbow Springs State Park: Sandhill Nature Trail (p. 231)

Best Hikes for Kids

3   Bivens Arm Nature Park (p. 42)

9   Morningside Nature Center (p. 74)

18   UF NATL Nature Trails (p. 126)

31   Carney Island Recreation & Conservation Area (p. 210)

36   Sholom Park (p. 237)

37   Silver Springs State Park: River Trails (p. 243)

Best Hikes for Scenic Vistas

Best Hikes for Seclusion

Best Hikes for Wildlife

Introduction

About This Book

Though polar opposites in many ways—hip, green college town versus retiree mecca—Gainesville and Ocala, only 35 miles apart, share a love of the outdoors. Student clubs from the University of Florida hike the same trails as Volksmarch groups from The Villages, enjoying wilderness immersion in the Ocala National Forest and scrambles on rugged terrain along the Cross Florida Greenway and in the hills of San Felasco Hammock. Centered on two counties—Alachua and Marion—along I-75 in North Central Florida, the region is both home base to the Florida Trail Association and the home of where the statewide Florida Trail began, the Ocala National Forest. Grassroots conservation, in the form of Pennies for Parks, helped preserve places near Ocala such as Rainbow Springs from development; aggressive land-conservation programs by Gainesville, Alachua County, and the nonprofit Alachua Conservation Trust have ensured that some of that area's most beautiful places are preserved for public access. This book is divided based on cities and land management: the Ocala National Forest, which lies to the east of both cities, has its own chapter, as does the Cross Florida Greenway, which crosses the state south of Ocala. Hikes nearest Gainesville are in the "Gainesville & Vicinity" chapter, and hikes nearest Ocala are in the "Ocala & Vicinity" chapter. No hike is more than 1.25 hours from the farther of the two city centers.

Gainesville & Vicinity

Bisected by I-75 and US 441, the city of Gainesville—the seat of Alachua County and home to the University of Florida—sits atop rolling hills with deeply forested ravines. This is an area defined by karst features, particularly sinkholes. Fed by seepage springs, Hogtown Creek rises at the north end of the city and flows

1

southwest, where a handful of nature parks provide access to the beautiful, clear, sand-bottomed waterway. It vanishes into a sinkhole near Lake Kanapaha. To the east of downtown lies cypress-lined Newnan's Lake, surrounded by a floodplain that drains, as Prairie Creek, toward Paynes Prairie. Sweetwater Creek, which flows right through downtown, also ends up in Paynes Prairie, and all of the waterways in Paynes Prairie vanish into the Alachua Sink. South of Paynes Prairie near Micanopy, a historic village established in 1821, are smaller prairies ringed with wetlands and old-growth oak hammocks. Rolling hills to the southeast and northwest of the city support upland habitats like pine flatwoods, sandhills, and North America's southernmost swath of eastern deciduous forest.

Ocala National Forest

When Theodore Roosevelt put pen to paper to designate the Ocala National Forest in 1909, it was the second national forest established east of the Mississippi River. Created to protect the world's largest sand pine scrub forest, known as the Big Scrub, it is a place of incredible natural wonders first described by William Bartram in his *Travels* in 1774. Home of many first- and second-magnitude springs amid a mosaic of open prairies, longleaf pine islands, and the desertlike scrub, it is bounded by the floodplains of the St. Johns River to the east and the Ocklawaha River to the west. It is a top destination for hikers and backpackers visiting Florida, with more than 100 miles of hiking available on dozens of trails, including the most popular portion of the statewide Florida National Scenic Trail. From these, we've selected our top picks for you.

Cross Florida Greenway

It was to be a deep ditch across Florida, envisioned by the first surveyors in Florida as a quick passage to the Gulf of Mexico, a route for commerce, America's own Panama Canal. It would have torn the state in two, and irreparably damaged the Flordian Aquifer. Work on the Cross Florida Barge Canal began in the 1930s to provide jobs during the Great Depression and continued in fits and starts through the late 1960s. Several decades after the project was abandoned—in no small part thanks to an active group of environmentalists wanting to protect the scenic beauty of the Ocklawaha River and Silver Springs—the lands were transferred to the state of Florida and became the Marjorie Harris Carr Cross Florida Greenway, Florida's first official greenway. A mile wide in most places, it hosts parallel hiking, mountain biking, and equestrian trail systems that meet at trailheads and at the Land Bridge over I-75.

Ocala & Vicinity

Known as the Horse Capital of the World, Ocala—the center of Marion County—is surrounded by hundreds of horse farms on hundreds of thousands of acres of rolling hills that parallel I-75. On its eastern side is Silver Springs, the community that grew up around one of the largest and deepest natural springs in the world; to the west, Dunnellon is the home of Rainbow Springs, another first-magnitude spring. An important military post during the 1820s—with Fort King the flashpoint for the Second Seminole War—Ocala made its mark as an agricultural mecca with orange groves and cattle ranches. Today, retirement communities have replaced ranches, with explosive growth down the FL 200 corridor paralleled by a portion of the Cross Florida Greenway. This region extends past Dunnellon to encompass hikes along the eastern edge in old-growth forests in Levy County, and south past Belleview to Lake Weir.

To select the 38 hikes profiled in this guide, we visited more than 50 trail systems and parks. Putting the hikes up against the five-star rating system (see Star Ratings, page 6) used for this series helped us narrow them down to the best. Scenery in Florida is subjective—we rarely have panoramic vistas along our trails, although a handful of those presented in this guidebook do. We gave high marks for scenery to trails where you could look around and feel a part of the landscape, where the habitats immerse you in the hiking experience

3

with few outside distractions. No hikes merit five stars in all of the ratings categories, of course, since some are weighted toward wilderness experiences and others toward ease of taking young children out on the trail.

How To Use This Guidebook

The following information walks you through this guidebook's organization to make it easy and convenient for planning great hikes.

Overview Map, Map Key, & Map Legend

The overview map on the inside front cover depicts the location of the primary trailhead for all 38 hikes described in this book. The numbers shown on the overview map pair with the map key on the inside front cover facing page. Each hike's number remains with that hike throughout the book. Thus, if you spot an appealing hiking area on the overview map, you can flip through the book and find those hikes easily by their sequential numbers at the top of each profile page.

Trail Maps

In addition to the overview map on the inside cover, a detailed map of each hike's route appears with its profile. On each of these maps, symbols indicate the trailhead, the complete route, significant features, facilities, and topographic landmarks such as creeks, overlooks, and peaks. A legend identifying the map symbols used throughout the book appears on the inside back cover.

To produce the highly accurate maps in this book, the authors used a handheld GPS unit to gather data while hiking each route, and then sent that data to the publisher's expert cartographers. However, your GPS is not a substitute for sound, sensible navigation that takes into account the conditions that you observe while hiking.

Despite the high quality of the maps in this guidebook, the publisher and authors strongly recommend that you always carry an additional map, such as the ones noted in each profile opener's "Maps" listing.

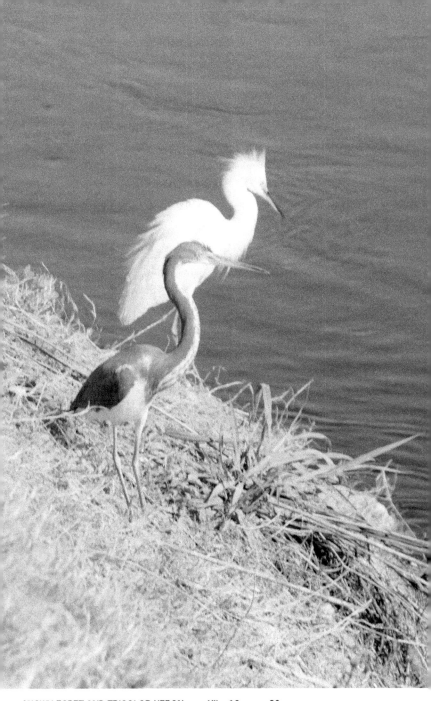

SNOWY EGRET AND TRICOLOR HERON; *see Hike 10, page 80*

The Hike Profile

Each profile opens with the hike's star ratings, GPS trailhead coordinates, and other key at-a-glance information—from the trail's distance and configuration to local contacts. Each profile also includes a map (see "Trail Maps," above). The main text for each profile includes four sections: Overview, Route Details, Nearby Attractions, and Directions (for driving to the trailhead area). Below is an explanation of each of those elements.

STAR RATINGS

Five-Star Trails is the title of a Menasha Ridge Press guidebook series geared to specific cities across the United States, such as this one for Gainesville and Ocala. Following is the explanation for the rating system of one to five stars in each of the five categories for each hike. Rankings are comparative to other trails in Florida.

FOR SCENERY:

★ ★ ★ ★ ★	Unique or picturesque panoramas
★ ★ ★ ★	Diverse vistas
★ ★ ★	Pleasant views
★ ★	Unchanging landscape
★	Not selected for scenery

FOR TRAIL CONDITION:

★ ★ ★ ★ ★	Consistently well maintained
★ ★ ★ ★	Stable, with no surprises
★ ★ ★	Average terrain to negotiate
★ ★	Inconsistent, with good and poor areas
★	Difficult to follow

FOR CHILDREN:

★ ★ ★ ★ ★	Babes in strollers are welcome
★ ★ ★ ★	Fun for anyone past the toddler stage
★ ★ ★	Good for young hikers with proven stamina
★ ★	Not enjoyable for children
★	Not advisable for children

FOR DIFFICULTY:

★ ★ ★ ★ ★   Grueling

★ ★ ★ ★   Strenuous

★ ★ ★   Moderate (won't beat you up—but you'll know you've been hiking)

★ ★   Easy with patches of moderate

★   Good for a relaxing stroll

FOR SOLITUDE:

★ ★ ★ ★ ★   Positively tranquil

★ ★ ★ ★   Spurts of isolation

★ ★ ★   Moderately secluded

★ ★   Crowded on weekends and holidays

★   Steady stream of individuals and/or groups

GPS TRAILHEAD COORDINATES

As noted in Trail Maps, above, the authors used a handheld GPS unit to obtain geographic data and sent the information to the publisher's cartographers. In the opener for each hike profile, the coordinates—the intersection of the latitude (north) and longitude (west)—will orient you from the trailhead. In some cases, you can drive within viewing distance of a trailhead. Other hiking routes require a short walk to the trailhead from a parking area.

You will also note that this guidebook uses the degree–decimal minute format for presenting the GPS coordinates. The latitude and longitude grid system is likely quite familiar to you, but here is a refresher, pertinent to visualizing the GPS coordinates:

Imaginary lines of latitude—called parallels and approximately 69 miles apart from each other—run horizontally around the globe. The equator is established to be 0°, and each parallel is indicated by degrees from the equator: up to 90°N at the North Pole, and down to 90°S at the South Pole.

Imaginary lines of longitude—called meridians—run perpendicular to latitude lines. Longitude lines are likewise indicated by degrees. Starting from 0° at the Prime Meridian in Greenwich, England, they continue to the east and west until they meet 180° later at the International Date Line in the Pacific Ocean. At the equator, longitude lines also are approximately 69 miles apart, but that distance narrows as the meridians converge toward the North and South Poles.

To convert GPS coordinates given in degrees, minutes, and seconds to the format shown above in degrees–decimal minutes, the seconds are divided by 60. For more on GPS technology, visit **usgs.gov.**

DISTANCE & CONFIGURATION

"Distance" notes the length of the hike round-trip, from start-to-finish. If the hike description includes options to shorten or extend the hike, those round-trip distances will also be factored in here. "Configuration" defines the trail as a loop, an out-and-back (taking you in and out via the same route), a figure eight, or a balloon.

HIKING TIME

A general rule of thumb for the hiking times noted in this guidebook is 2 miles per hour, with up to 2.5 miles an hour on easier trails. That pace allows time for taking photos, dawdling and admiring views, and alternating stretches of ascents and descents. When deciding whether to follow a particular trail in this guidebook, consider your own pace, weather, general physical condition, and energy level that day, as well as the description of the terrain along the route. In areas prone to flooding, expect no better than 1 mile an hour if you have to wade.

HIGHLIGHTS

Unique geologic or botanical features, historic sites, or other features that draw hikers to this trail are emphasized here.

ELEVATION

You will note that we have not listed elevation readings in the key information that introduces each hike, nor have we included any elevation profiles. The highest point in the state of Florida is documented to be the Panhandle's Britton Hill, at 345 feet. Thus, we decided that including elevation in this book was not necessary to help you plan or engage in hiking in Gainesville and Ocala.

ACCESS

Fees or permits required to hike the trail are detailed here—and noted if there are none. Trail-access hours are also shown here.

MAPS

Resources for maps, in addition to those in this guidebook, are listed here. (As previously mentioned, the publisher and authors recommend that you carry more than one map and that you consult those maps before heading out on the trail in order to resolve any confusion or discrepancy.)

FACILITIES

Alerts you to restrooms, picnic tables, campgrounds, playgrounds, and other facilities at or near the trailhead.

WHEELCHAIR ACCESS

Tells you if there are paved sections or other areas that can safely accommodate a wheelchair.

COMMENTS

Here you will find assorted nuggets of information, such as whether dogs are allowed on the trails.

CONTACTS

Listed here are phone numbers and websites for checking trail conditions and other details.

OVERVIEW, ROUTE DETAILS, NEARBY ATTRACTIONS, & DIRECTIONS

These four elements provide the main text about the hike. "Overview" gives you a quick summary of what to expect on that trail; the "Route Details" guide you on the hike, start-to-finish; "Nearby Attractions" suggests appealing area sites, such as restaurants, museums, and other trails. "Directions" will get you to the trailhead from a well-known road or highway.

Weather

October–April is the best time for hiking around Gainesville and Ocala, with fall and spring the best seasons to enjoy magnificent wildflowers. It's always a joy when the first frost comes along, since it means the insects won't trouble us for a couple of months. As the heat and humidity can be intense and rains fall heavily during the summer months—when afternoon thundershowers are the norm—summer hiking should start soon after sunrise and be completed before noon. For trails in this region that traverse floodplains: if there has been rain recently in the area, check ahead regarding flooding to avoid having to wade through a trail.

The following chart lists average temperatures and precipitation by month for the Gainesville/Ocala area. For each month, "Hi Temp" is the average daytime high; "Lo Temp" is the average nighttime low; and "Rain" is the average precipitation.

MONTH	HI TEMP	LO TEMP	RAIN
January	71°F	42°F	3.3"
February	75°F	45°F	3.3"
March	79°F	50°F	4.5"
April	84°F	68°F	2.6"
May	90°F	62°F	2.9"
June	92°F	69°F	7.4"
July	93°F	71°F	6.9"
August	93°F	72°F	6.3"
September	91°F	69°F	6.0"
October	85°F	62°F	3.0"
November	79°F	51°F	2.1"
December	73°F	44°F	2.5"

Water

How much is enough? In Florida, the humidity tricks you into thinking you don't need to drink more water, when in fact you do. A hiker walking steadily in 90° heat needs approximately 10 quarts (2.5 gallons) of fluid per day. We carry a minimum of a quart for every 4 miles we hike, and double that when the temperatures rise above 80°. It's always smart to hydrate before your hike and make sure you have water in your car when you return to the trailhead to hydrate some more. For most people, the pleasures of hiking make carrying water a relatively minor price to pay to remain safe and healthy. So pack more water than you anticipate needing, even for short hikes.

If you are tempted to drink surface water, do so with extreme caution. Agricultural runoff can be an issue in this region. Swamp water teems with little creatures. Even those pretty springs in pristine areas can host parasites. Drinking such water presents inherent risks for thirsty trekkers. Giardia parasites contaminate many water sources and cause the dreaded intestinal giardiasis that can last for weeks after ingestion. For information, visit The Centers for Disease Control website at **cdc.gov/parasites/giardia.**

Effective treatment is essential before using any water source found along the trail. Boiling water for 2–3 minutes is always a safe measure for camping, but day hikers can consider iodine tablets, approved chemical mixes, filtration units rated for giardia, and UV filtration. Some of these methods (for example, filtration with an added carbon filter) remove bad tastes typical in stagnant water, while others add taste. As a precaution, carry a means of water purification to help in a pinch if you realize you have underestimated your consumption needs. A water-purifying straw is a lightweight emergency option you can keep at all times in your day pack.

Clothing

Weather, unexpected trail conditions, fatigue, extended hiking duration, and wrong turns can individually or collectively turn a great outing into an uncomfortable one at best—and a life-threatening one at worst. Thus, proper attire plays a key role in staying comfortable and, sometimes, in staying alive. Here are some helpful guidelines:

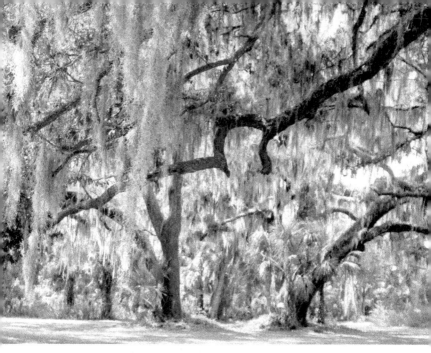

ANCIENT OAKS ON CARNEY ISLAND; *see Hike 31, page 210*

- ★ Choose silk, wool, or synthetics for maximum comfort in all of your hiking attire, from hats to socks. Cotton is fine if the weather remains dry and stable, but you won't be happy if that material gets wet.

- ★ Always wear a hat, or at least tuck one into your day pack or hitch it to your belt. Hats offer all-weather sun and wind protection as well as warmth if it turns cold.

- ★ Be ready to layer up or down as the day progresses and the mercury rises or falls. Today's outdoor wear makes layering easy, with such designs as jackets that convert to vests and zip-off or button-up legs.

- ★ Wear running shoes, hiking boots, or sturdy hiking sandals with toe protection. Flip-flopping along a paved urban greenway is one thing, but never hike a trail in open sandals or casual sneakers. Your bones and arches need support, and your skin needs protection.

- ★ Pair that footwear with good socks. If you prefer not to sheathe your feet when wearing hiking sandals, tuck the socks into your day pack; you may need them if you get tired of sand between your toes.

- ★ Rain gear is an absolute must in Florida, even if the day starts out clear and sunny. Tuck into your day pack, or tie around your waist, a jacket that is breathable and either water-resistant or waterproof.

Essential Gear

What's in your pack? The following list includes never-hike-without-them items, in alphabetical order, as all are important:

★ *Extra food* (trail mix, granola bars, or other high-energy foods)

★ *First-aid kit,* personalized to your needs

★ *Flashlight or headlamp* with extra bulb and batteries

★ *Insect repellent,* especially in summer (Spray beforehand, too.)

★ *Map and compass or GPS.* If you use a GPS, always remember to take a data point where your car is parked so you can find it again. Spare batteries are a must, too.

★ *Sunglasses*

★ *Sunscreen* (Note the expiration date on the tube or bottle; it's usually embossed on the top.)

★ *Water* (As emphasized more than once in this book, bring more than you think you will drink. Depending on your destination, you may want to bring a container of chemical treatment or a filter for purifying water in case you run out.)

★ *Whistle* (This little gadget will be your best friend in an emergency.)

First-Aid Kit

In addition to the items above, those below may appear overwhelming for a day hike. But any paramedic will tell you that the products listed here—in alphabetical order, because all are important—are just the basics. The reality of hiking is that you can be out for a week of backpacking and acquire only a mosquito bite—or you can hike for an hour, slip, and suffer a bleeding abrasion or broken bone. Fortunately, these items collapse into a very small space. You may also purchase a convenient prepackaged kit at your pharmacy or online.

★ Ace bandages or Spenco joint wraps

★ Antibiotic ointment (Neosporin or the generic equivalent)

★ Athletic tape

★ Band-Aids

★ Benadryl or the generic equivalent diphenhydramine (*in case of allergic reactions*)

★ Blister kit (such as Moleskin or Spenco 2nd Skin)

★ Butterfly-closure bandages

★ Epinephrine in a prefilled syringe (typically by prescription only, for people known to have severe allergic reactions to hiking occurrences such as bee stings)

★ Gauze (one roll and a half dozen 4-by-4-inch pads)

★ Hydrogen peroxide or iodine

★ Ibuprofen or acetaminophen

Note: Consider your intended terrain and the number of hikers in your party before you exclude any article cited above. A walk in an urban park or on a very short nature trail may not inspire you to carry a complete kit, but anything beyond that warrants precaution. When hiking alone, you should always be prepared for a medical need. And if you are hiking with a friend or with a group, one or more people in your party should be equipped with first-aid material.

General Safety

The following tips may have the familiar ring of your mother's voice.

★ *Always let someone know where you will be hiking and how long you expect to be gone.* It's a good idea to give that person a copy of your route, particularly if you are headed into any isolated area. Let them know when you return.

★ *Always sign in and out of any trail registers provided.* Don't hesitate to comment on the trail condition if space is provided; that's your opportunity to alert others to any problems you encounter.

★ *Do not count on a cell phone for your safety.* Reception may be spotty or nonexistent on the trail, even on an urban walk—especially if it is under heavy tree cover. Most carriers have *no* cell phone service in the center of the Ocala National Forest.

★ *Always carry food and water, even for a short hike.* And bring more water than you think you will need. (This cannot be said often enough.)

★ *Ask questions.* Forest rangers and park employees are there to help. It's a lot easier to solicit advice before a problem occurs, and it will help you avoid a mishap away from civilization.

★ *Stay on designated trails.* Even on the most clearly marked trails, there is usually a point where you have to stop and consider in which direction to head. If you become disoriented, don't panic. As soon as you think you may be off track, stop, assess your current direction, and then retrace your steps to the point where you went astray. Using a map, a compass, and this book, and keeping in mind what you have passed thus far, reorient yourself, and trust your judgment on which way to continue. If you become absolutely unsure of how to continue, return to your vehicle the way you came in. Should you become completely lost and have no idea how to find the trailhead, remaining in place along the trail and waiting for help is most often the best option for adults and *always* the best option for children.

★ *Always carry a whistle,* another precaution that cannot be overemphasized. It may be a lifesaver if you do become lost or sustain an injury.

★ *Be especially careful when wading into water.* Whether you are fording a stream or sloshing across a flooded trail, make every step count. If you have any doubt about maintaining your balance, use a trekking pole or stout stick for balance. If the water seems too deep to wade, turn back. Whatever is on the other side is not worth risking your life.

★ *Be careful along shorelines, bluffs, and the rims of deep sinkholes.* While these areas may provide spectacular views, they are potentially hazardous. Stay back from the edge of bluffs, and make absolutely sure of your footing; a misstep can mean a nasty and possibly fatal fall. Even when covered in a tangle of vines and cypress knees, shorelines of rivers and marshes may have alligators and snakes sunning along them.

★ *Standing dead trees and storm-damaged living trees pose a significant hazard to hikers.* These trees may have loose or broken limbs that could fall at any time. While walking beneath trees, and when choosing a spot to rest or enjoy your snack, look up.

★ *Know the symptoms of subnormal body temperature known as hypothermia.* Shivering and forgetfulness are the two most common indicators of this stealthy killer. Yes, hypothermia can occur in Florida, even in the summer, especially when the hiker is wearing lightweight cotton clothing that gets wet. If symptoms present themselves, get to shelter, hot liquids, and dry clothes as soon as possible.

★ *Know the symptoms of heat exhaustion (hyperthermia).* Lightheadedness and loss of energy are the first two indicators. If you feel these symptoms, find some shade, drink your water, remove as many layers of clothing as practical, and stay put until you cool down. Marching through heat exhaustion leads to heatstroke, which can be fatal. If you should be sweating and you're not, that's the signature warning sign. Your hike is over at that point—heatstroke is a life-threatening condition that can cause seizures, convulsions, and eventually death. If you or a companion reaches that point, do whatever can be done to cool the victim down, and seek medical attention immediately.

★ *Most important of all, take along your brain.* A cool, calculating mind is the single most important asset on the trail. It allows you to think before you act.

★ *In summary:* Plan ahead. Watch your step. Avoid accidents before they happen. Enjoy a rewarding and relaxing hike.

Watchwords for Flora & Fauna

ALLIGATORS Alligators are the number one fear that new hikers to Florida have. But we'll take an alligator stretched across a trail over a grizzly any day. Alligators are rarely a threat to humans, unless they've been fed and associate you with a food source. That means when you're hiking, you should never, ever throw your food scraps into or near a body of water. Pack them out or get a friend to eat the leftovers. It also means being careful where you hike with a dog. Never bring a dog along—especially a small one—if you're hiking into a swampy area. Some of the hikes in this book are especially dangerous for dogs, with warnings posted at the trailheads to leave your dog behind. Believe them.

Most alligators move out of your way when they hear you coming. But if an alligator is on the footpath and refuses to move after you've made a lot of noise—banging a hiking stick on the ground might help—don't walk up close to it. Give it a wide berth, circling around its tail end so it doesn't feel trapped or threatened. If you're out at the end of the La Chua Trail (Hike 10) and can't get back to the trailhead because a big, sullen gator is blocking your way and won't move, it's time to call the park ranger for help. This hike has more alligators per square foot than any other one in Florida.

BITING FLIES When a deerfly or a horsefly bites, it feels like a chunk of your skin is being gouged out. Yellow flies, which lurk in deeply shaded areas, go for the head and shoulders and can drive you right off the trail. During unusually wet seasons, black flies emerge in small numbers, eager to harass. Covering your skin and using liberal amounts of insect repellent are your best means of protection. Even then, you'll still probably get bitten. All of these flies appear during the summer months, another reason why we prefer to hike any other time of year in Florida.

BLACK BEARS Although no one has ever been attacked by a Florida black bear, the sight or approach of a bear can give anyone a start. If you encounter a bear while hiking, remain calm and avoid running in any direction. Make loud noises to scare off the bear, and back away slowly. In primitive and remote areas, assume bears are present— they are common in the Ocala National Forest, for instance, and throughout the Silver River basin. In more developed sites, check on the current bear situation prior to hiking. Most encounters are food related, as bears have an exceptional sense of smell and not particularly discriminating tastes. While this is of greater concern to backpackers and campers, on a day hike, you may plan a lunchtime picnic or munch on a snack from time to time. So remain aware and alert.

MOSQUITOES Mosquitoes, as you'd imagine, grow bigger here in Florida, and there are 80 different species just waiting to harass you. They're not just a summer occurrence—we've been bitten in the middle of December in a warm year. Mosquitoes are primarily found in deeply shaded areas and are worst at sunrise and sunset. Ward them off with insect repellent and/or repellent-impregnated clothing. In some areas of Florida, mosquitoes are known to carry the West Nile virus, so all due caution should be taken to avoid their bites.

POISON IVY, OAK, & SUMAC Recognizing and avoiding poison ivy, oak, and sumac are the most effective ways to prevent the painful, itchy rashes associated with these plants. Poison ivy occurs as a vine or ground cover, three leaflets to a leaf, and is commonly encountered in hardwood hammocks and floodplain forests. Sometimes the vines, which can climb well up into the canopy on tree trunks, grow so large that the leaves can be mistaken for hickory leaves up above you. Poison oak also has three leaflets. Poison sumac flourishes in swampland, each leaf having 7–13 leaflets. Urushiol, the oil in the sap of these plants, is responsible for the rash. Within 14 hours of exposure, raised lines and/or blisters will appear on the affected area, accompanied by a terrible itch. Refrain from scratching, because bacteria under your fingernails can cause an infection. Wash and dry the affected area thoroughly, applying a calamine lotion to help dry out the rash. If itching or blistering is severe, seek medical attention. If you do come into contact with one of these plants, remember that oil-contaminated clothes, hiking gear, and pets can easily cause an irritating rash on you or someone else, so wash not only any exposed parts of your body but also any exposed clothes, gear, and pets.

SNAKES Florida has only six species of venomous snakes, five of which are found in this region: pygmy rattlesnake, eastern diamondback rattlesnake, timber rattlesnake, cottonmouth, and coral snake. Rattlesnakes like to bask in the sun and won't bite unless threatened. Cottonmouths are extremely territorial and will stand their ground.

The snakes you most likely will see while hiking are non-venomous species and subspecies, with black snakes and rat snakes being the most common. The best rule is to leave all snakes alone, give them a wide berth as you hike past, and make sure any hiking companions (including dogs) do the same.

When hiking, stick to well-used trails, and wear over-the-ankle boots and loose-fitting long pants. Do not step or put your hands beyond your range of detailed visibility, and avoid wandering around in the dark. Step *onto* logs and rocks, never *over* them, and be especially careful when climbing rocks. Always avoid walking through dense brush or saw palmetto thickets.

TICKS Ticks are often found on brush and tall grass, where they seem to be waiting to hitch a ride on a warm-blooded passerby. Adult ticks are most active October through May, paralleling hiking season. Among the varieties of ticks, the black-legged tick, commonly called the deer tick, is the primary carrier of Lyme disease. Wearing light-colored clothing makes it easier for you to spot ticks before they migrate to your skin. At the end of the hike, visually check your hair, the back of your neck, your armpits, and your socks. During your post-hike shower, take a moment to do a more complete body check. For ticks that are already embedded, removal with tweezers is best. Use disinfectant solution on the wound.

Hunting

Separate rules, regulations, and licenses govern the various hunting types and related seasons. Though there are generally no problems, hikers may wish to forgo trips during general gun season (deer season) in late fall and early winter, when the woods suddenly seem filled with orange and camouflage, especially in the Ocala National Forest. For specific hunting season dates on public lands, visit the Florida Fish & Wildlife Conservation Commission website: **myfwc.com.**

Regulations

Regulations vary among land management agencies throughout the region, with additional regulations piled onto some lands that are jointly managed by county and water management districts. Always check the trail kiosk when you arrive at a trailhead, as additional rules may apply. The following agencies adhere to certain regulations year-round.

ALACHUA CONSERVATION TRUST

★ No ATVs or motorized vehicles.

★ No littering, dumping, or smoking.

★ No removal or disturbance of plants, animals, or artifacts.

★ No hunting or shooting.

ALACHUA COUNTY LAND CONSERVATION DIVISION

★ For your own safety, stay on the trail.

★ No dogs permitted where posted.

★ Where permitted, dogs must be leashed.

★ Pack out what you pack in.

★ Where cyclists are permitted, bikers must yield to hikers.

★ Leave what you find. Collecting plants, animals, artifacts, or fossils is prohibited.

★ Visitors who remain after posted hours are trespassing.

CITY OF GAINESVILLE PARKS AND RECREATION

An extensive list of regulations is part of the city code found at **bit.ly/gnvparkregs.** These are some highlights:

★ Motorized vehicles remain in parking areas.

★ Where permitted, dogs remain on leash and on trail.

★ Plants, animals, and cultural resources remain undisturbed.

★ Litter and pet waste are placed in appropriate containers.

★ Foot traffic and bikes remain on trails.

★ Do not feed, release, or remove animals.

★ Alcohol and firearms are prohibited.

★ Smoking and ground fires are prohibited due to wildfire risk.

FLORIDA STATE FORESTS

★ Primitive camping requires a permit in advance and a fee.

★ Hunting or fishing requires a valid Florida license, available from the Florida Fish & Wildlife Conservation Commission.

FLORIDA STATE PARKS

★ Day-use hours are generally 8 a.m.–sunset.

★ Dogs must be leashed.

★ Hunting is not permitted.

★ Fishing, where permitted, requires a valid Florida fishing license, available from the Florida Fish & Wildlife Conservation Commission.

★ Fishing, boating, swimming, and fires allowed in designated areas only.

★ Alcoholic beverage consumption is allowed in designated areas only.

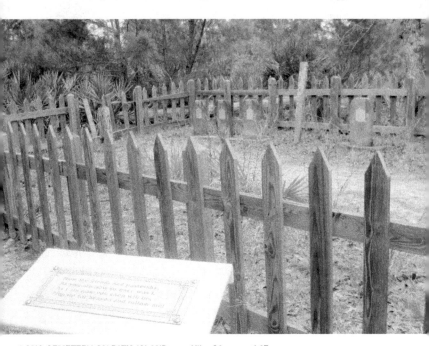

LONG CEMETERY ON PAT'S ISLAND; *see Hike 21, page 145*

★ All plants, animals, and park property are protected. The collection, destruction, or disturbance of plants, animals, or park property is prohibited.

MARION COUNTY PARKS AND RECREATION

★ Dogs are generally prohibited, except at Marshall Swamp and Brick City Adventure Park. Where permitted, dogs must be leashed.

★ Prior authorization is needed for the placement of geocaches or the use of metal detectors.

★ Marion County residents with 100% disabilities and active-duty military personnel are eligible to receive one complimentary annual park pass.

OCALA NATIONAL FOREST

A comprehensive list of rules and regulations is available on the Ocala National Forest website, **www.fs.usda.gov/ocala.** These are a few highlights:

★ You are responsible for your own safety.

★ Leave natural areas the way you find them.

★ Do not block, restrict, or interfere with the use of roads or trails.

★ Do not damage or remove any historic or archaeological resource.

★ Pets must always be restrained or on a leash while in developed recreation sites.

★ Throw all garbage and litter in containers provided for this purpose, or take it with you.

ST. JOHNS WATER MANAGEMENT DISTRICT

A full list of recreational rules, along with information on wheelchair and mobility-device access, may be found at **sjrwmd.com/recreation /usinglands.html.** These are some highlights.

★ Each individual is responsible for determining his or her personal ability to access District trails safely.

★ Fishing, where permitted, requires a valid Florida fishing license.

★ Hiking, jogging, bird-watching or any other activity where travel is by foot only is allowed on District lands except in areas restricted by signs.

★ Dogs, cats, or other domestic animals, excluding horses, are allowed on District land provided that they are leashed at all times.

★ Removal of plants, animals, or archeological or cultural resources is not allowed.

Trail Etiquette

Always treat the trail, wildlife, and fellow hikers with respect. Here are some reminders.

★ Plan ahead in order to be self-sufficient at all times. For example, carry necessary supplies for changes in weather or other conditions. A well-planned trip brings satisfaction to you and to others.

★ Hike on open trails only.

★ In seasons or construction areas where road or trail closures may be a possibility, use the websites or phone numbers listed for each hike to check conditions prior to heading out. Do not attempt to circumvent such closures.

★ Avoid trespassing on private land, and obtain all permits and authorization as required. Leave gates as you found them or as directed by signage.

★ Be courteous to other hikers, bikers, equestrians, and others you encounter on the trails.

★ Never spook wild animals or pets. An unannounced approach, a sudden movement, or a loud noise startles most critters, and a surprised animal can be dangerous to you, to others, and to itself. Give animals plenty of space.

★ Observe the yield signs around the region's trailheads and backcountry. Typically they advise hikers to yield to horses, and bikers to yield to both horses and hikers. When encountering mounted riders on shared trails, hikers can courteously step off the trail. So the horse can see and hear you, calmly greet the riders before they reach you, and do not dart behind trees. Also resist the urge to pet horses unless you are invited to do so.

★ Stay on the existing trail and do not blaze any new trails.

★ Be sure to pack out what you pack in, leaving only your footprints. No one likes to see the trash someone else has left behind.

Tips on Hiking around Gainesville and Ocala

For a pleasant outdoor experience, plan your hikes between October and April. Take along a field guide—the *National Audubon Society Field Guide to Florida* is a good general guide—to learn about the plants and animals you encounter along the trail. Our website, **floridahikes .com**, contains detailed information on habitats along Florida's trails and specific identifications of some of the common wildflowers, trees, and birds mentioned in this book, as well as information for planning hikes throughout Florida. You'll also find photo galleries so you can sample the trails before you hike, as well as GPX downloads for the trails in this book.

Avoid traveling on major highways during weekday rush hours. Traffic is especially heavy on I-75 in Gainesville in the mornings and evenings. FL 200 in Ocala near I-75 turns into a parking lot some afternoons. Many of the hikes in this book are along scenic back roads, and we encourage you to use those to traverse the region in a more relaxed manner.

Hikes located in floodplain areas may be under water after a heavy rain or a generally rainy season. Before you head out for any of the hikes within floodplain basins, you can determine if the trails are flooded based on notices of river levels at the St. Johns Water Management District website: **sjrwmd.com.**

This book includes some of the most scenic (and easiest to day hike) segments of the statewide Florida Trail, a 1,400-mile National Scenic Trail, in this region. It's one of only two National Scenic Trails in America that traverse a single state. While a handful of people thru-hike the trail each year, many more enjoy it on day hikes and backpacking trips along sections strung across the state, from Big Cypress National Preserve near Naples to Gulf Islands National Seashore in Pensacola.

The statewide Florida Trail Association brings together volunteers to build and maintain trail sections: **floridatrail.org.**

On weekends, urban parks and parks that are popular camping destinations get very busy. Some parks, like Juniper Springs Recreation Area, close their gates when their parking areas reach capacity. This can happen early on Saturday mornings. If you have your heart set on doing a certain hike on a certain Saturday, get there early.

While most of the hikes in the book have no entrance fee, those in Florida State Parks do. If you're a frequent parks traveler, consider purchasing an annual pass, good throughout the entire Florida State Parks system, now numbering more than 160 parks: **floridastateparks.org/thingstoknow/annualpass.cfm.**

The City of Gainesville Parks and Recreation Department, Nature Operations Division, has many more nature parks to explore. Many have no on-site parking and can only be reached on foot from nearby neighborhoods or bus stops. The department offers guided tours of some of its harder-to-access public lands: **natureoperations .org.** Similarly, Alachua County Forever offers "open by appointment" tours of its public lands that aren't accessible except on a walk with a biologist: **alachuacounty.us.**

Marion County Parks and Recreation charges entrance fees for its most popular county parks. An annual park pass is available to Marion County residents: **marioncountyfl.org.**

Entrance fees are often charged for public lands managed by Florida State Forests, including Goethe State Forest. An annual pass is available: **floridaforestservice.com.**

Frequent guided hikes are offered throughout the region by volunteers with the Florida Crackers Chapter of the Florida Trail Association. Going with a group is a fun way to meet fellow hikers and learn more about other outdoor activities in the area. See Appendix C for details.

Gainesville and Vicinity (Hikes 1–19)

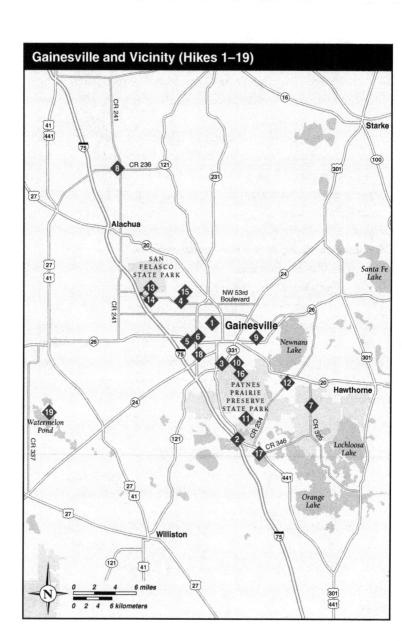

Gainesville & Vicinity

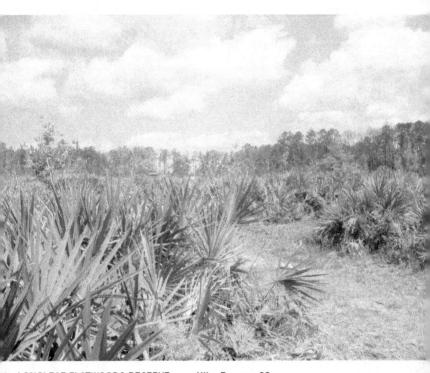

LONGLEAF FLATWOODS RESERVE; *see Hike 7, page 62*

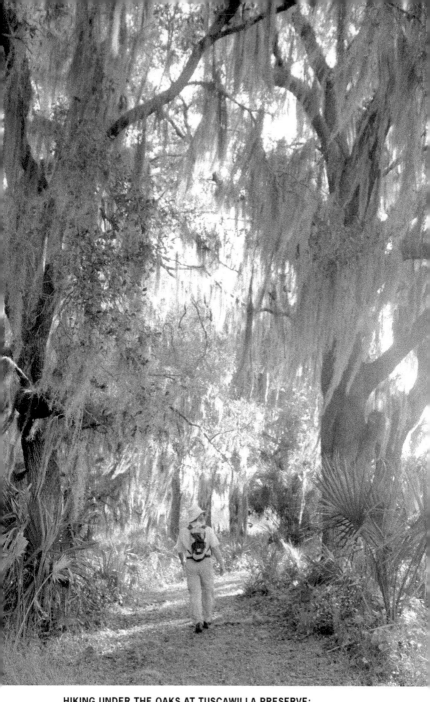

HIKING UNDER THE OAKS AT TUSCAWILLA PRESERVE;
see Hike 17, page 122

Alfred A. Ring Park

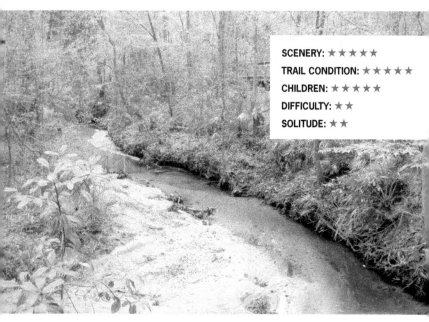

SCENERY: ★ ★ ★ ★ ★
TRAIL CONDITION: ★ ★ ★ ★ ★
CHILDREN: ★ ★ ★ ★ ★
DIFFICULTY: ★ ★
SOLITUDE: ★ ★

HOGTOWN CREEK

GPS TRAILHEAD COORDINATES: N29° 40.455' W82° 20.815'

DISTANCE & CONFIGURATION: 1.5-mile out-and-back with loop

HIKING TIME: 1 hour

HIGHLIGHTS: Scenic, hilly terrain above Hogtown Creek; ancient trees; spring wildflowers

ACCESS: November–April: daily, 8 a.m.–6 p.m. May–October: daily, 8 a.m.–8 p.m. Free.

MAPS: USGS *Gainesville East,* on trailhead kiosk

FACILITIES: Restrooms and water fountain adjoining playground, benches along the trail, informational kiosks at all entry points, detailed interpretive information

WHEELCHAIR ACCESS: Possible on boardwalk and level terrain above the creek; use NW 16th Avenue (southern entrance) as entry point (no parking available at this entrance).

COMMENTS: Pets welcome. Primary access and parking is on the grounds of the Elks Club. Please use the designated spaces for park visitors.

CONTACTS: City of Gainesville Department of Parks, Recreation and Cultural Affairs, Nature Operations Division: 352-334-5067; **natureoperations.org; facebook.com/cityof gainesvillenature**

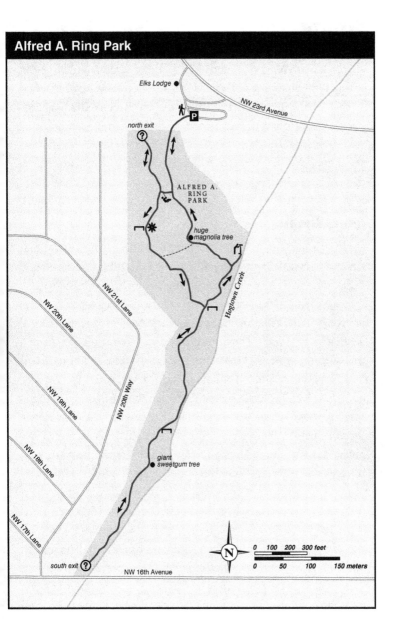

Alfred A. Ring Park

Elks Lodge

NW 23rd Avenue

north exit

ALFRED A.
RING PARK

huge
magnolia tree

Hogtown Creek

NW 21st Lane

NW 20th Lane

NW 19th Lane

NW 20th Way

NW 18th Lane

giant
sweetgum tree

NW 17th Lane

south exit

NW 16th Avenue

N

0   100 200 300 feet
0   50   100   150 meters

Overview

Alfred Ring knew the value of forests. Leaving Germany for America six years after World War I ended, he put himself through college and came to the University of Florida in 1947 to teach, eventually serving as chair of the department of real estate and land studies. His textbooks on land valuation sold more than 10 million copies. By donating a strip of dense slope forest with old-growth trees and rare wildflowers along Appalachian-style ravines, he allowed the City of Gainesville to open Alfred A. Ring Park as its first linear nature park in 1990.

Route Details

Leaving the parking area, you descend toward a broad iron bridge that stretches across Hogtown Creek, a gateway into this popular nature park. From there, it's a climb into the upland forest on a broad natural footpath. Skinny loblolly pines tower overhead. You come to an interpretive sign, "Discover the Habitats of Ring Park," that gives an introduction to what you're about to see. At the top of the hill, you reach a trail junction in front of the restrooms, playground, and picnic pavilion. Turn right to walk uphill through the forest, where you'll notice dogwood blooming in late winter. You reach the north entrance to the park at a kiosk, which has a map of the trail system. Come back along the same path to the playground, and turn right to walk through this hub of activity, where moms gather with their tots. On the other side, the trail enters the pretty Emily S. Ring wildflower garden, with native plants—including silver-tinged saw palmetto— accompanied by colorful azalea and camellia. A bench sits in front of a goldfish pond.

The trail descends out of the cultivated wildflower garden into the upland forest. In spring the hillside is carpeted with smooth Solomon's seal, a wildflower identified with the southern Appalachians. Were it not for the bluestem palms along the slope, you'd think you were hiking in the Appalachians on the steep descent to the creek. Passing a trail junction, continue straight ahead and downhill into the slope forest, where massive Southern magnolias cast broad pools of shade.

At a half mile, the trail reaches a T intersection with a trail paralleling the creek. Turn right to follow this route downstream. A bench overlooks a pretty horseshoe curve in the creek, just before you start walking down a broad boardwalk. As the waters of Hogtown Creek ebb and flow—based on not just rainfall but also stormwater pushed into it from surrounding subdivisions—it casts up sandy beaches along the natural curves of the stream. Along the boardwalk, you see one of the giant stormwater pipes peeking out of a deeply eroded side channel feeding the creek. The valley created by erosion over time sustains a lush slope forest. Needle palms glisten along the water's edge, and red buckeye thrives in the deep shade cast by enormous specimens of Florida maple, sweetgum, bluff oak, and loblolly pine. Substantial boardwalks provide overlooks of the many lazy bends of the creek in its deeply folded basin.

The trail comes up to a fence with a well-established neighborhood and jogs left along another boardwalk. The large shaggy-barked tree you pass is a swamp chestnut oak with enormous leaves. This type

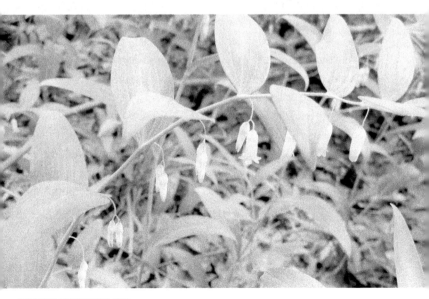

SMOOTH SOLOMON'S SEAL

of oak thrives in places where limestone outcrops close to the surface, as it does here in Gainesville. The karst geology means that Hogtown Creek doesn't end its journey into a lake or river; it simply vanishes into a big sinkhole at the south end of the city at a preserve called Split Rock Conservation Area.

At the next boardwalk, you'll pass a loblolly pine of impressive stature. Watch for poison ivy, which curls around tree trunks and sneaks up to the edges of the well-groomed footpath. Look up, too, to see how the tall, thin loblolly pines curve skyward through the forest canopy. As the creek continues its sinuous path through the forest, the footpath connects a string of benches and boardwalks. Squirrels scramble through the stands of tall, thin loblolly pines and play balance beam over the clear waters of Hogtown Creek as they dash across fallen logs.

When you hear traffic, you've reached the southern pedestrian entrance to Alfred A. Ring Park at NW 16th Avenue. This is your turnaround point, at 0.8 mile. Walk back the way you came, following Hogtown Creek upstream. With the ravine to your right, you'll notice many more wildflowers down the steep slope. By 1.2 miles you reach the trail junction with the bench where you started this trek along the ravine. Continue straight, where a sign indicates this is the direction to the observation deck and parking area.

As the trail works its way through a flatter floodplain, you can see a water-filled depression, a sink, to the right and obvious side channels carved when the creek is in flood stage. Just past the trail junction is an observation deck with interpretive information about the floodplain of Hogtown Creek. The creek is off to the right, more slender and steeply sided, with a tiny cascade pouring in from a tributary. As you exit the observation deck, turn right and start the gentle climb. You encounter a strange habitat transition along this part of the trail, with bracken fern—which likes dry places—growing closer to the creek, and netted chain—which likes dampness—growing farther up the slope. In a lush slope forest, an interpretive sign explains

34

some of the rarer plants that can be spotted here, like the cranefly orchid and Florida spiny pod, as well as basswood and wild azalea.

At the trail junction, turn right. Towering over the forest on the left is one of the largest Southern magnolias you may ever see, with a trunk that rises at least 50–60 feet before the first branches reach out above the canopy. It's not the only oversized Southern magnolia here; you walk between rows of them as the trail slowly rises up to meet the trail junction at the restrooms. Turn right to exit. As you descend to the bridge, you're more aware of the sheer size of the trees of this forest, especially the magnolias nearest the creek. Crossing the bridge, continue to the parking area to finish this 1.5-mile hike.

Nearby Attractions

This is the closest hike to Gainesville's renowned outfitter, Brasingtons Adventure Outfitters: **brasingtons.com.** Hiking trails upstream at 29th Road Nature Park provide another perspective on the creek; Hogtown Creek Headwaters (not open at the time of our research) lets you see the source of the beautiful creek that flows through Alfred A. Ring Park: **natureoperations.org.**

Directions

From I-75, Exit 390, take FL 222 east for 4.3 miles to FL 121 (NW 34th Boulevard). Turn right. Make the first left onto NW 31st Avenue. Follow this road 1.2 miles to the traffic circle; continue around it and straight onto NW 31st Avenue. Follow the curve of the road to the right as it becomes NW 23rd Boulevard. The park entrance is on the right, inside the parking area for the Elks Lodge. Address: 1800 NW 23rd Boulevard.

2 # Barr Hammock Preserve

SCENERY: ★ ★ ★ ★ ★
TRAIL CONDITION: ★ ★ ★ ★ ★
CHILDREN: ★ ★
DIFFICULTY: ★ ★
SOLITUDE: ★ ★

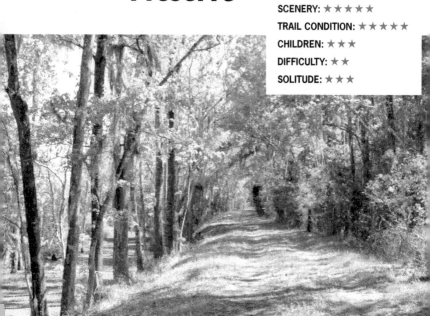

ALONG THE SHADED SOUTH LEVEE

GPS TRAILHEAD COORDINATES: N29° 30.973' W82° 18.363'

DISTANCE & CONFIGURATION: 6.8-mile loop

HIKING TIME: 2.75 hours

HIGHLIGHTS: Extensive views across Levy Prairie, great birding

ACCESS: Daily, sunrise–sunset. Free.

MAPS: USGS *Micanopy*, on trailhead kiosk and available at kiosk

FACILITIES: Trailhead kiosk, benches

WHEELCHAIR ACCESS: The levee has natural surfaces with some rough and grassy spots and some grades. However, a wheelchair cannot fit through the stile.

COMMENTS: Pets prohibited for your safety and theirs. The trail is shared with cyclists. Take plenty of water, as more than half of the trail has no shade, and wear sunscreen and a hat. Please heed the cautions about leaving the levee. Alligators and snakes may sun on the footpath. Watch out for fire ant nests and holes in the levee.

CONTACTS: Alachua County Environmental Protection Department, Land Conservation Division: 352-264-6800; **alachuacounty.us**

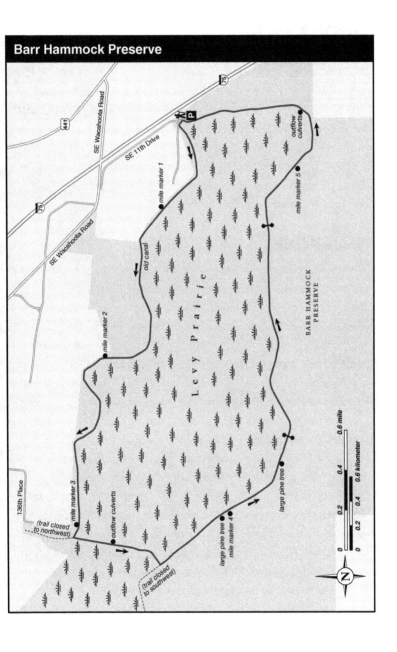

Barr Hammock Preserve

Overview

Encompassing more than 5,700 acres, Barr Hammock Preserve includes an expansive wetland area, the Levy Prairie, which is the centerpiece of the Levy Loop Trail, literally. Entirely atop a set of levees, the Levy Loop Trail rings the broad expanse of this wet prairie west of Micanopy. The trailhead, off Wacahoota Road, adjoins the west side of I-75 with ample parking and a kiosk with maps. No other trails are in place at this time, although there appears to be plenty of room to expand the trail system, with 25 miles of trails described in the management plan for the preserve.

Route Details

Walk through the pass-through stile and stay to the right at the trail junction to walk counterclockwise around the loop starting with the North Levee, which lets you tackle the side of the trail with no shade first. The sweep of Levy Prairie will be to your left for the duration of the hike. In this broad open space, wind rushes across the water, generating a nice swamp-cooler effect off the marsh. To the right, the floodplain is covered in water spangles, with Virginia willow, red maple, and elderberry rising from the edges.

When you see the first warning sign, it will make you laugh. The preserve managers don't want you to step off this levee, and they tell you why, with some comical drawings. Heed their advice. After a quarter mile, the trail—which is broad enough for trucks to drive on—turns a corner to the right, revealing the vastness of the Levy Prairie. The wetlands around you are full of life, with frogs croaking, evidence of gator slides, and lots of bird chatter. At a half mile you see something really strange-looking on the right, like a giant rock; it turns out to be gigantic sculpture in front of an even bigger home, next to cabbage palms just beyond the boundary of the wetlands. A handful of homesteads hide behind the trees to the right. Passing a pasture on the right, where cows may be browsing, the trail makes a sharp left, heading away from the shoreline and out into the prairie on the levee. You see what looks like an old canal bisecting the wetlands. Just beyond it, there is a little bit of open water. The paralleling canal is where the fill for the levee came from.

By 1.1 miles a pretty prairie stretches to the shoreline, a bluff densely shaded by live oaks with an understory of saw palmetto. Passing marker 2, which indicates it is 1.5 miles back to the trailhead, the levee hugs close to the rim of the prairie, with just a small wetland between you and the treeline. Dog fennel and sea myrtle block your views along one stretch. Cypresses crowd the prairie rim near a yard with a deer feeder. As the trail curves away from the rim again, there are larger trees on the right, obscuring the view. Passing small signs that say CONSERVATION EASEMENT at the base of the dike, you can smell the deep, thick mud. Sand cordgrass grows in clumps in the shallow wetlands. The prairie rim is a pretty mix of live oaks and cabbage palms, recalling the scenes that William Bartram described as he explored this area in 1774.

Past another mileage marker, the trail comes to a junction with a sign that says TRAIL CLOSED at 2.7 miles. Turn left to continue around the Levy Prairie. Watch for alligators, as there is an active alligator slide right after this turn. The dike becomes a straightaway through the heart of the prairie. Up ahead is a forest, offering the promise of hiking in shade. Before you reach it, the trail crosses culverts with manual valves enabling the movement of water from the larger prairie into the lower prairie on the right. You see an island topped with cabbage palms and a handful of oaks, mostly dead and ghostly-looking in their shrouds of Spanish moss. Flanked by canals on both sides, the trail begins to enter the forest.

You reach another TRAIL CLOSED sign as the trail comes to a T intersection at 3.2 miles, adjoining an outflow culvert that releases water out of the prairie and into the floodplain forest. Turn left to start your walk down the South Levee, a shady corridor along the remains of an old fence with weathered wooden posts. The canal on the left is covered in water spangles, obscuring the water, and on the right is a tannic stream flowing away from the prairie into a gum swamp. In breaks between the trees, you can look out across the sweep of Levy Prairie. A towering loblolly pine on the left has three trunks, each topped with its own distinct crown the size of a large pine tree.

At 4 miles the trail jogs left and faces another long straight-away. You'll find this pattern repeated for most of the remainder of the hike, with the trail on the South Levee mainly in the shade of older trees. Many of the loblolly pines along this part of the trail are of significant size, along with a mammoth-sized sugar hackberry and some monstrous poison ivy vines growing in proportion to these big trees. Down on your right, the habitat transitions to a blackwater swamp, where royal ferns cast reflections against the dark, sluggish water. Passing through an old gate—this was most recently a cattle ranch, with a fence dropping down into the soggy prairie grasses—the trail continues to provide sweeping views across the prairie, with the best panoramas from this next section. At one point, you can see most of the entire route of the hike that you've followed thus far.

As vegetation begins to obscure the views, an old levee goes off to the left into a weedy area just as the trail curves to the right down another long straightaway. You see water lilies in patches of open water. Although there are many trees atop the levee, shade is at more of a premium. Wading birds congregate in shallow pools along the prairie's edge. Through the leafy floodplain forest to the right, you start to see a flash of speeding cars in the distance as the trail draws closer to I-75. Crossing another gator slide, the trail passes through the next old gate at 5.4 miles. Look at the barbed wire fence on the right; it's been consumed by the ever-growing girth of a large oak tree.

Losing elevation, the levee drops down to meet the level of both wetlands that flank it, making this an easy place for alligators to scramble between them or sun on the trail. The path curves to the right to enter a shady straightaway. The sound of peeping frogs fills the air. Several species are known to frequent the preserve, including spring peepers and Florida cricket frogs. Passing the next mile marker at 5.7 miles, the trail remains close to the wetlands and then rises up again. You see tall slash pines on the right as the habitat transitions from gum swamp to an island of pine flatwoods. Crossing an outflow culvert, where cattails rise out of the pool of water above the floodgates, the outflow from Levy Prairie feeds the next gum swamp.

The trail jogs left down another straightaway, providing one last view of the open prairie at 6.4 miles. Royal fern clusters at the base of the levee. You know you're getting close to the end of the loop as the traffic noise from I-75 keeps getting louder. Ending the loop, turn right to exit through the stile, completing a 6.8-mile hike.

Nearby Attractions

Established in 1821, the historic town of Micanopy feels like a step back in time. Look for antiques and art within the beautiful buildings along the main thoroughfare, Cholokka Boulevard: **micanopychamber .com.** Surrounded by beautiful gardens, the Herlong Mansion provides an elegant place to stay: **herlong.com.** The main entrance to Paynes Prairie Preserve State Park, where you'll find the Wacahoota Trail (Hike 11) and other trails, is along US 441: **floridastateparks.org /paynesprairie.**

Directions

From I-75, Exit 374, Micanopy, drive east on CR 234 toward US 441. Turn north on US 441 and continue 1 mile to Wacahoota Road. Turn left and drive 0.6 mile, crossing over I-75 on an overpass. Take the first left—a sharp, doubling-back left—after the overpass onto Southeast 11th Drive. Continue down this sometimes-bumpy dirt road for 0.6 mile. It ends at the trailhead.

Bivens Arm Nature Park

SCENERY: ★ ★ ★ ★
TRAIL CONDITION: ★ ★ ★ ★ ★
CHILDREN: ★ ★ ★ ★
DIFFICULTY: ★ ★
SOLITUDE: ★

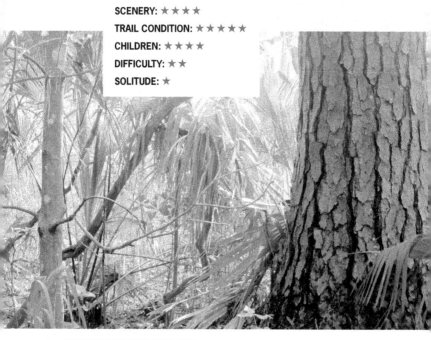

ANCIENT PINE AT BIVEN'S ARM

GPS TRAILHEAD COORDINATES: N29° 37.200' W82° 19.939'

DISTANCE & CONFIGURATION: 1.5-mile loop

HIKING TIME: 30 minutes

HIGHLIGHTS: Birding at the willow marsh, ancient live oak hammock, wildflowers

ACCESS: Daily, 8 a.m.–5 p.m. Gate closes after 5 p.m. Free.

MAPS: USGS *Micanopy,* on trailhead kiosk

FACILITIES: Restrooms and picnic pavilion adjoining playground, benches along the trail, informational kiosks at trailhead, large pavilion overlooking marsh

WHEELCHAIR ACCESS: Along boardwalk and paved paths at the start of the trail system

COMMENTS: Pets prohibited. The paths are great for kids, but don't let them run ahead of you. There are natural hazards such as poison ivy and the potential of alligators near the marsh edge.

CONTACTS: City of Gainesville Department of Parks, Recreation and Cultural Affairs, Nature Operations Division: 352-334-5067; **natureoperations.org**; **facebook.com/cityof gainesvillenature**

Bivens Arm Nature Park

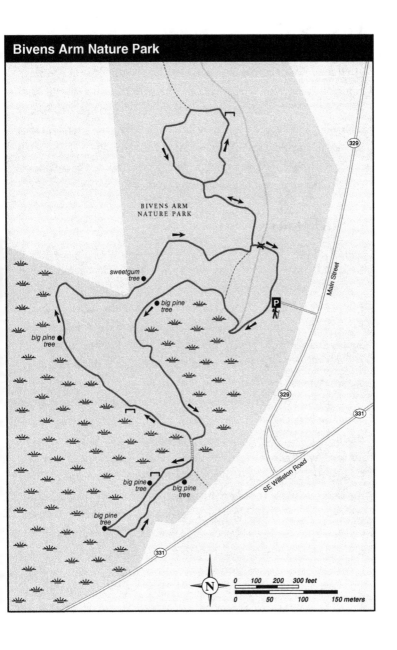

BIVENS ARM
NATURE PARK

sweetgum
tree

big pine
tree

big pine
tree

P

big pine
tree

big pine
tree

big pine
tree

329

331

Main Street

329

331

SE Williston Road

N

| 0 | 100 | 200 | 300 feet |
| 0 | 50 | 100 | 150 meters |

Overview

Providing a firsthand look at how water makes its way through southern Gainesville to Paynes Prairie, Bivens Arm Nature Park lies between some of Gainesville's busiest roads. Water trickles through the landscape in small streams from Colobaugh Pond, Tumblin Creek, and drainage ditches from as far away as the University of Florida campus to feed this marshy watershed, which in turn flows into Paynes Prairie. Protecting these forests and marshes since 1981, the park features some of the largest pines and live oaks you'll see in the area.

Route Details

Start your hike at the kiosk. Just beyond is the junction of a boardwalk and a paved path going off to the right. Walk straight ahead toward the willow marsh, where you'll see a warning sign: DO NOT FEED THE ALLIGATORS. This pretty marsh is the heart of Bivens Arm, the connector between Bivens Arm Lake to the northwest and Paynes Prairie to the south. The Gary R. Junior Pavilion provides an easy place for birders to scan the marsh. Although traffic noise is persistent, there is always birdsong here.

Leaving the pavilion, start down the boardwalk, which crosses East Tumblin Creek. The boardwalk follows the edge of the marsh through an oak and pine forest. At boardwalk's end, you reach a trail junction with another caution sign about alligators; here they can wander up onto the footpath. Turn left at this junction and go down the ramp to follow the footpath along the edge of the marsh. Southern magnolia and large sand live oaks dominate this stretch of forest, and the footpath is very rooty underfoot. Poison ivy is prevalent in the understory, and smilax vines form huge heaps. Magnolia leaves crunch underfoot as you walk.

At a quarter mile an extraordinarily twisted loblolly pine is along the trail, hanging out over the marsh near where an old trail has been closed off. Straight ahead is the Gator Gap Loop Trail. Cinnamon fern shows up in the damp places between the footpath and the marsh. A short side path leads to a collection of cypress knees poking out of the edge of the swamp. Back on the main trail, you walk under an arched limb that drops straight down and into the ground on the other side of the trail. You just can't get away from the traffic noise at this end of the park, but the setting is quite beautiful.

Coming to a trail junction after 0.4 mile, turn left and cross a boardwalk across a sluggish creek. Turn right to start a loop. The trail drops toward the floodplain, more willow marsh with red maples on its edge. A bench is set in the perfect spot to look at a dogwood in bloom. Draperies of Spanish moss glisten in the sunlight in the oak canopy. Past an enormous pine, the trail curves into the heart of the oak hammock on the return loop. At the T intersection, turn left to complete this loop, returning to the boardwalk and trail junction. Continue straight ahead. Passing the base of another large slash pine, the trail turns right, following the edge of the willow marsh. At 0.7 mile a bench faces the wetland under the shade of large live oaks.

Large live oaks arch overhead, shading the footpath. The trail winds its way through an area dappled with sunlight, where several large trees have fallen, and passes a side trail on the left to an apartment

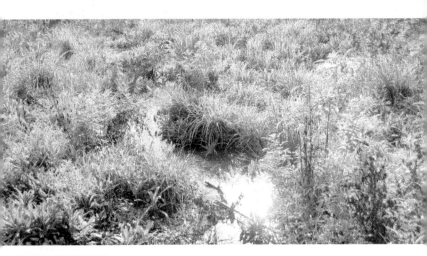

BIVEN'S ARM MARSH

complex. Meandering through denser forest, it reaches the trail junction with the boardwalk that led you into the trail system. Turn left. The next junction comes up quickly, within sight of a small bridge. Turn left again. You'll pass a marker designating this area the Kirkwood Addition, the newest part of the park and the best area for wildflowers.

Smooth Solomon's seal thrives in this well-shaded upland along East Tumblin Creek. Zebra longwing butterflies flit between the big oaks, alighting on red buckeye growing near a stand of yaupon holly. You reach the fork in the trail, the bottom of this loop, after 1.2 miles. Keep left. Devil's walking stick grows along the footpath's edge, which enters a forest with more towering loblolly pines. Southern magnolia fills the middle canopy. At the next fork, keep to the right, passing a bench near a short cabbage palm. The trail begins a downward trend, losing elevation as it heads back toward the creek. As you reach the end of the loop, turn left.

At the junction, turn left to take the bridge over Little Tumblin Creek, which leads to a paved sidewalk. Passing a gigantic American holly next to the picnic pavilion, the path turns right and leads you under the arch of a live oak limb back to the parking area, completing this 1.5-mile hike.

Nearby Attractions

Just up Main Street, Gainesville's vibrant downtown district includes many distinctive and popular restaurants: **visitgainesville.com/down town.** The Top, a retro-themed haven for fusion comfort food, is one of our favorites. The hip place for live theater is the Hippodrome Theater: **thehipp.org.**

Directions

From I-75, Exit 382, drive east on Southeast Williston Road (FL 331) for 2.7 miles. After you cross US 441, get in the left lane. Take the next left onto Main Street. Drive up to the first U-turn spot, past the park entrance, to come back downhill and enter the park on the right.

Devil's Millhopper
Geological State Park

SCENERY: ★ ★ ★ ★ ★
TRAIL CONDITION: ★ ★ ★ ★ ★
CHILDREN: ★ ★ ★
DIFFICULTY: ★ ★ ★ ★
SOLITUDE: ★ ★

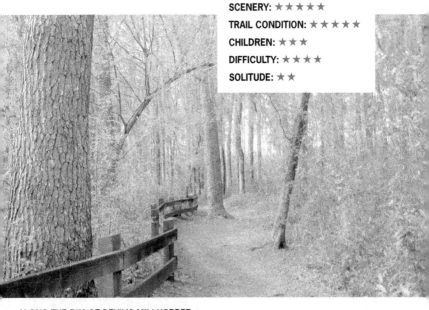

ALONG THE RIM OF DEVIL'S MILLHOPPER

GPS TRAILHEAD COORDINATES: N29° 42.341' W82° 23.685'

DISTANCE & CONFIGURATION: 0.9-mile balloon

HIKING TIME: 45 minutes

HIGHLIGHTS: Waterfalls, rugged terrain, uncommon wildflowers

ACCESS: Wednesday–Sunday, 8 a.m.–5 p.m. Entrance fee: $2 per pedestrian or cyclist; $4 per car.

MAPS: USGS *Gainesville West,* at visitor center

FACILITIES: Restrooms and visitor center at the trailhead, many benches along the nature trail and staircase

WHEELCHAIR ACCESS: The loop trail around the sinkhole is a natural-surface footpath but very firm. The bottom of the sinkhole can be viewed at the visitor center.

COMMENTS: Leashed dogs welcome. Every Saturday at 10 a.m., a park ranger leads a guided walk.

CONTACTS: Devil's Millhopper Geological State Park: 352-955-2008; **floridastateparks.org/devilsmillhopper**

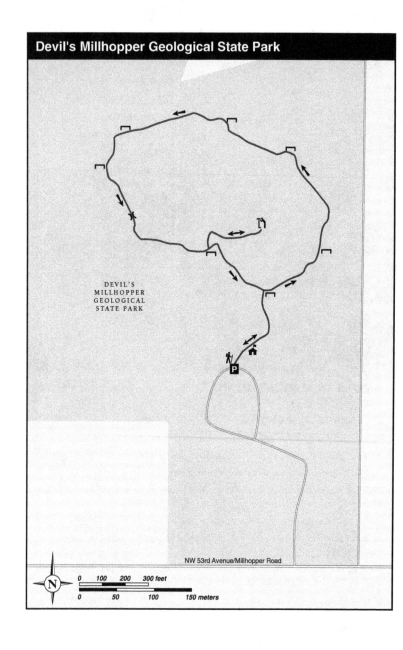

Devil's Millhopper Geological State Park

DEVIL'S
MILLHOPPER
GEOLOGICAL
STATE PARK

NW 53rd Avenue/Millhopper Road

N

0   100   200   300 feet

0   50   100   150 meters

Overview

Though this hike is short, you're going in deep: 236 steps lead to the bottom of Devil's Millhopper, a massive sinkhole that breaks up the karst landscape of northern Gainesville. Karst is eroded limestone bedrock, a landform where sinkholes and caves and underground streams are the norm. Although this geological site is one of many deep sinkholes found throughout Florida on public lands, its long history as a tourist attraction and the fact that waterfalls cascade inside its walls at certain times of the year make it a major draw.

Route Details

From the parking area, follow the paved path up to an open-sided 1970s visitor center, which has restrooms and a theater showing a short film under the roof. Behind the visitor center, walk straight down the walkway toward the sinkhole to meet the nature trail loop. Turn right, passing a bench. The massive tree on your left is a spruce pine, which loves limestone. It has a very dark bark and tiny pinecones like a sand pine. If it's just rained a day or two before, you can hear the echo of waterfalls inside the sinkhole. When you look left, you can see the enormity of this big hole in the ground, more than 500 feet across.

By 0.2 mile you pass a bench on the right with an unobstructed view of the sinkhole. A low fence parallels the trail on the sinkhole side, as the bluff drops off steeply. Passing another enormous spruce pine—this time with an interpretive marker—the trail continues under a canopy of large slash pines, Southern magnolia, and a variety of oaks, including a swamp chestnut oak. By a bench, you see a double-trunked slash pine that does a twist around itself. Shiny blueberries grow in the understory as the habitat transitions into scrubby flatwoods.

The trail makes a sharp left to enter an upland forest. At 0.5 mile you cross a bridge over a deep Appalachian-style ravine, with Carolina basswood, American holly, and tall loblolly pines and blue-jack oaks rising from its slopes. The trail turns left to parallel the ravine. Cedars cluster around a clearing where the staircase descends into the sinkhole.

And now it's down, down, down the stairs into the depths of the Devil's Millhopper, a 120-foot drop in elevation. As water from the ravine percolates through a series of small waterfalls, you hear the constant cascade over the tumble of limestone boulders that fill this passage. The staircase provides great views directly over the flow. In earlier times, visitors scrambled down the slopes—a dangerous proposition—until a path was built to the bottom in later years. You can see a remnant of that steep path along one of the turns in the staircase, at an interpretive sign: "Trails Old and New."

At the bottom of the sinkhole, the staircase becomes a board-walk leading you past more cascades and a sinuous creek that vanishes out of sight into the karst below. At certain times of year, you

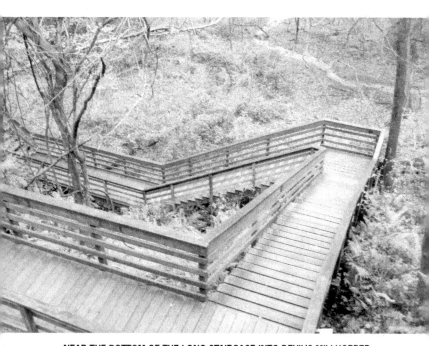

NEAR THE BOTTOM OF THE LONG STAIRCASE INTO DEVIL'S MILLHOPPER

can see tall, slim waterfalls, like you'd see in Hawaii, falling down the far wall of the sinkhole. These are fed by a perched water table. Boardwalk's end is at an observation platform with a needle palm nearby and a waterfall upslope. Since all of this movement of water is entirely dependent on rainfall and overall seasonal conditions, there are times you may visit and only see a dribble of water. No worries; it's a short trail. Come back again after a rain.

The downside of climbing down a huge staircase is the walk back up. As you rest along the landings, take the time to peer over the railing and look for unusual wildflowers. Near the old trail into the sinkhole, a jack-in-the-pulpit thrives below a rock overhang. The drop in temperature as you descend into the sinkhole creates a cool microclimate where plants you'd normally only find farther north, including trillium, can survive.

Reaching the top of the sinkhole and level ground again, take a moment to check out the monument recognizing Devil's Millhopper as a registered National Natural Landmark since 1976. This site became a Florida State Park in 1974. Turn left to exit, passing the restrooms and visitor center en route to the parking area to wrap up this 0.9-mile walk.

Nearby Attractions

Kids and adults alike will enjoy the Santa Fe Teaching Zoo at Santa Fe College: **sfcollege.edu/zoo.** San Felasco Park (Hike 15) sits directly north, and the hiking trails of San Felasco Hammock Preserve State Park (Hikes 13 and 14) are 4.2 miles west along Millhopper Road.

Directions

From I-75, Exit 390, take FL 222 east 3.4 miles to NW 43rd Street. Turn left. Continue 1 mile north to Millhopper Road and turn left. Devil's Millhopper Geological State Park is on your right.

John Mahon Nature Park

SCENERY: ★ ★ ★ ★
TRAIL CONDITION: ★ ★ ★ ★ ★
CHILDREN: ★ ★ ★ ★ ★
DIFFICULTY: ★ ★
SOLITUDE: ★

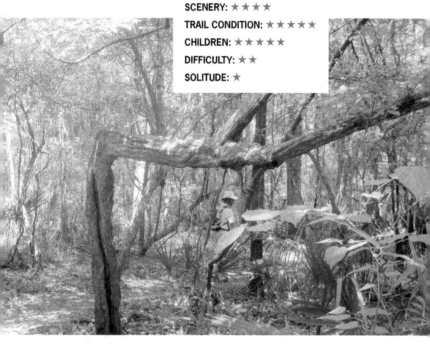

HIKING THROUGH DENSE HARDWOOD HAMMOCK

GPS TRAILHEAD COORDINATES: N29° 39.162' W82° 23.220'

DISTANCE & CONFIGURATION: 0.5-mile balloon

HIKING TIME: 20 minutes

HIGHLIGHTS: Uncommon wildflowers, beautiful hydric hammock, birding

ACCESS: Daily, sunrise–sunset. Free. No parking permitted after sunset.

MAPS: USGS *Gainesville West,* on trailhead kiosk

FACILITIES: Kiosk and picnic tables at trailhead, benches and interpretive stations along the trail

WHEELCHAIR ACCESS: None

COMMENTS: Pets welcome. Watch for poison ivy along the edges of the trail. Access to the park is also possible from the adjoining neighborhood if the lot at LifeSouth is full.

CONTACTS: City of Gainesville Department of Parks, Recreation and Cultural Affairs, Nature Operations Division: 352-334-5067; **natureoperations.org**; **facebook.com/cityof gainesvillenature**

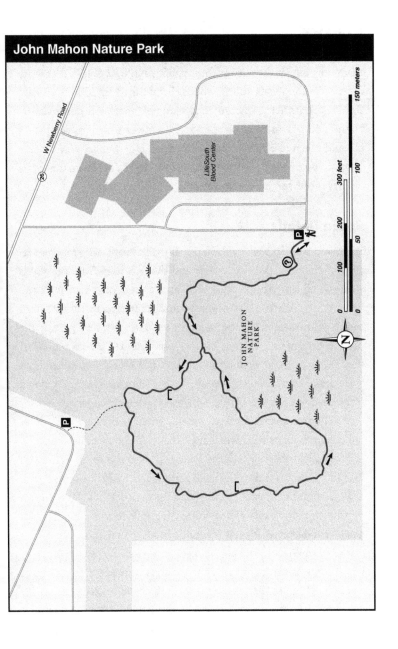

Overview

Ten acres isn't a lot of land for a nature park, but in this urban setting along one of the busiest thoroughfares in Gainesville, it's plenty for a refreshing walk in the woods. Established in 2006 with help from residents in the adjacent Sugarfoot neighborhood, John Mahon Nature Park is an oasis of deep shade between medical complexes on land donated by a medical consortium. One side faces Newberry Road, but you can't see the traffic for the trees. The name honors a history professor and conservationist who lived nearby.

Route Details

Start your walk by visiting the kiosk at the park entrance for an overview of the natural communities and the trail map. The trail starts adjacent to the picnic tables and, past a sign that says NATURE SANCTUARY, starts a slow descent through pines to an upland mixed forest with water oak, hickory, and sweetgum forming part of the canopy. Smilax and Virginia creeper send tendrils across the forest floor, with poison ivy intermingled in the greenery. Brilliant red trumpet honeysuckle dangles in clusters from vines draping down from the oaks. The footpath is broad and well maintained.

The trail swings out into a sunny corridor flanked by a wall of tall trees providing a screen against the traffic you can hear rushing past along Newberry Road. Stepping back into the shade again, you reach a fork in the trail as the habitat shifts to a hydric hammock with dozens of bluestem palms rising from the dark earth. Keep right. An interpretive sign explains the palms and their habitat. The forest is dense and deeply shaded as you come to a bench with a plaque honoring Susan Wright, who helped make this park a reality. Thick grapevines, some as thick as a tree trunk, dangle from the high canopy of oaks. Traffic noise increases as you climb uphill, where you can see a parking area through the vegetation on the right—for the other medical complex that flanks this preserve; a side trail leads to it at 0.2 mile. Continue past it and stay on the main trail.

Pay attention to the forest floor around you, as the deep shade offers less-common wildflowers, including sundial lupine, green dragon, and trillium, a place to thrive. The landscape slopes left, rolling down into a lower elevation where water collects beneath the tall oak trees. As you turn your back on the traffic sounds of Newberry Road, the trail descends into deeper shade. Passing the next bench, the trail continues to descend. You see a devil's walkingstick with its unique geometric pattern of leaves, then the trail curves to the left and keeps dropping downhill. There are a few houses on the right just beyond the screen of forest.

The trail makes a right past an unusual musclewood tree with a trunk bent at a right angle. Soon after, you see bluestem palms ahead, marking the end of this short but scenic loop. Continue straight ahead, following the trail on its gradual ascent through the upland mixed forest as it curves right and climbs back up to the trailhead, completing this half-mile hike.

Nearby Attractions

Clear Lake Nature Park can be reached by a walk through the adjoining neighborhood, and on the opposite side of Newberry Road toward the Oaks Mall, Cofrin Nature Park has trails through upland forests along Beville Heights Creek: **natureoperations.org.** You're not far from Loblolly Woods Nature Park (Hike 6) and the UF Cultural Complex, home to the UF NATL Nature Trails (Hike 18) and the Florida Museum of Natural History with its beautiful Butterfly Rainforest: **flmnh.ufl.edu.**

Directions

From I-75, Exit 387, Newberry Road, drive east past the Oaks Mall and continue toward the University of Florida. The park's address is 4300 Block W. Newberry Rd. A park sign on Newberry Road directs you to the south but doesn't make it obvious where you should park your car. Turn into the LifeSouth blood bank's parking lot. There are four designated parking spaces set aside in the back corner of this medical complex.

Loblolly Woods Nature Park

SCENERY: ★ ★ ★ ★ ★
TRAIL CONDITION: ★ ★ ★ ★
CHILDREN: ★ ★ ★ ★ ★
DIFFICULTY: ★ ★
SOLITUDE: ★ ★

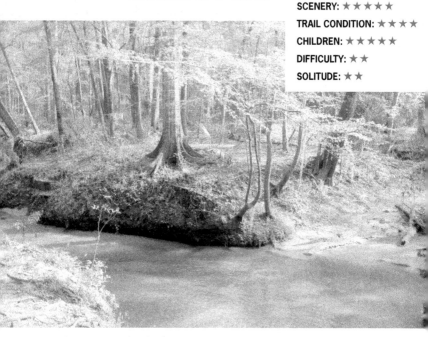

HOGTOWN CREEK IN LOBLOLLY WOODS

GPS TRAILHEAD COORDINATES: N29° 39.307' W82° 22.311'

DISTANCE & CONFIGURATION: 1.5-mile triple loop

HIKING TIME: 45 minutes

HIGHLIGHTS: Big trees, spring wildflowers, beautiful views of the creeks

ACCESS: Daily, sunrise–sunset. Free.

MAPS: USGS *Gainesville East,* on trailhead kiosk

FACILITIES: Restrooms at trailhead, benches along the trails

WHEELCHAIR ACCESS: Well-graded natural surface on the Hogtown Creek Greenway.

COMMENTS: Pets welcome. On weekends, expect to meet mountain bikers on the narrow trails in the woods. On the greenway, you'll always meet cyclists, but the path is broad and is the only part of the trail system suitable for strollers. Be cautious of poison ivy along the narrow side trails. The trail system continues north of NW 8th Avenue but is primarily used by local residents.

CONTACTS: City of Gainesville Department of Parks, Recreation and Cultural Affairs, Nature Operations Division: 352-334-5067; **natureoperations.org**; **facebook.com /cityofgainesvillenature**

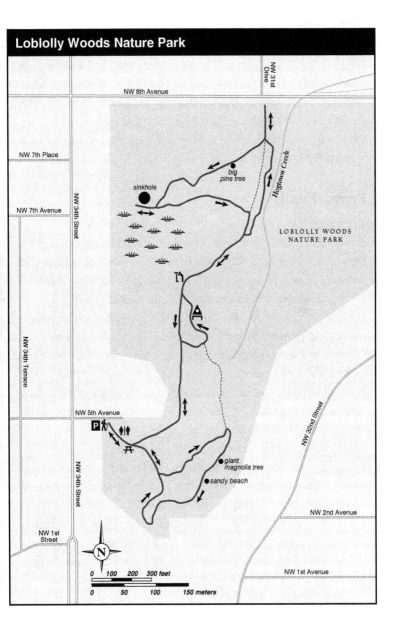

Loblolly Woods Nature Park

NW 31st Drive

NW 8th Avenue

NW 7th Place

NW 34th Street

big
pine tree

sinkhole

Hogtown Creek

NW 7th Avenue

LOBLOLLY WOODS
NATURE PARK

NW 34th Terrace

NW 5th Avenue

NW 32nd Street

NW 34th Street

giant
magnolia tree

sandy beach

NW 2nd Avenue

NW 1st
Street

N

NW 1st Avenue

| 0 | 100 | 200 | 300 feet |
| 0 | 50 | 100 | 150 meters |

Overview

An urban forest surrounded by the bustle of Gainesville, Loblolly Woods Nature Park protects 159 acres along the confluence of Possum Creek and Hogtown Creek. Spring wildflowers carpet the forest floor, and the namesake loblolly pines are some of the largest in the region. Bisected by a broad path long known as the Hogtown Creek Greenway, it's a place where narrow side trails lead to pretty bluffs above the creeks and sinkholes.

Route Details

Leaving the parking area, walk up the path past the former environmental center and a picnic bench at the entrance to the park. This broad path is the Hogtown Creek Greenway, a linear connector that gets a lot of use. Where you see fences that look like a gateway ushering you down a side trail, turn right. The trail approaches a small sinkhole in this dense bluff forest, where dogwoods bloom in late winter. There are lots of roots underfoot.

At a T intersection in the trail, a bluff overlooks the fast-moving water; you see the ripple effect in the sand bottom of the basin. The trail to the left was marked closed during our visit. Turn right and work your way down to the water's edge to cross the creek. At the top of the far bluff, keep left at the fork to follow the yellow blazes, simple dots on the trees, down a well-worn path. Sizable loblolly pines tower overhead. The trail passes a massive Southern magnolia with a split trunk. On the left is a sweeping sand bluff created by floodwaters depositing sand on a curve of the creek. You hear the burble of small rapids as you continue along the trail, finding smooth Solomon's seal in shady spots on the forest floor. The trail follows another bend in the creek, deeply carved from water rushing through a narrows around a horseshoe bend. You can walk out onto the horseshoe and see the meander of the creek around it. It's obvious that when it rains, floodwaters tear through this floodplain, reshaping the creek and its banks.

At the next trail junction, keep left. You start to see buildings beyond the trees as the trail reaches a peninsula near the residential and commercial district intersection of University Avenue and 34th Street. Follow the footpath as it curves to the right along the other waterway, merging into the blue triangle–blazed trail. Keep uphill at the fork, with the creek to your left, and stay left again at the junction of the yellow and blue trails, scrambling over a mass of roots. Reaching your original stream crossing after 0.4 mile, cross it again— it's easier to do from this direction, using the limestone and roots as steps—and return to the Hogtown Creek Greenway. Turn right.

This broad path tunnels through the forest. You'll see the first interpretive marker along this trek, on the layers of the forest, before another side trail at a fence tempts you back into the wilds of Loblolly Woods. There are more enormous Southern magnolias in this part of the woods, filling the air with sweet fragrance when they bloom in late May. When you reach a T intersection above the creek, turn left

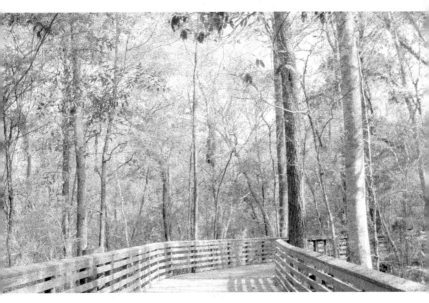

BOARDWALK ALONG THE HOGTOWN CREEK GREENWAY

to follow it, passing another sandy beach on an elbow in the creek. Sphagnum moss covers the banks of a narrow point in the creek. A loblolly pine with a split trunk towers over the trail. Resurrection fern swarms over oak limbs, lush and green after an evening's rain.

The trail follows the creek upstream to a bench at a beauty spot. You can sit along the creek here and listen to it burble. The trail guides you away from the creek and toward a break in the fence back to the greenway. Turn right. An observation deck is on the left. It's a place to look out over a large willow marsh, which is fed by spillover from the creek during its flood stage. You see tall pines off in the distance on its fringe, and elms and maples along this shoreline.

Leaving the observation deck, turn left to walk along the boardwalk, where there is a clump of needle palm at its far end. Just past it is another side trail for a walk down to the creek. Masses of small-leaf spiderwort, an invasive ground cover, blanket the slope. Turn left to follow the creek upstream. Grapevines grow very large here, as do many of the pines. Soft sand slopes down to the water. You can see the floodplain nature of the creek, the sand on the far bluffs carved as if with a knife. Another gap in the fence leads up to the greenway, but you can continue following the water's edge, being mindful of roots and vines.

Traffic noise signals the edge of the park. Turn left and walk up to the next gap in the fence to rejoin the greenway. It comes to a kiosk at NW Eighth Avenue, an alternate way to access Loblolly Woods if you couldn't find parking at the main entrance. At 0.9 mile this is your turnaround point. Peek down the street and you'll see large models of the planets lining the sidewalk.

Returning along the Hogtown Creek Greenway, take the next trail on the right into the forest, passing a patch of woodland phlox. Flanked by native bamboo, the footpath leads you to the largest of the loblolly pines along the trail so far. A big swale next to the trail is dry but can fill with floodwaters when the creek is high. The trail curves around this swale, coming within sight of a water-filled sinkhole surrounded by dense forest. Large live oaks arch over the pathway.

Turn right at the next T intersection, and walk down a little ways to see the sink more closely. The trail ends at a fence. Turn around and backtrack under the big oaks, walking past the trail junction, along a natural levee between the floodplain swale and willow marsh. Reaching a gap in the Hogtown Creek Greenway fence at 1.2 miles, turn right and start walking back along the greenway. You'll cross the boardwalk again and pass the observation deck, taking the more direct route back through the woods to the trailhead to complete the 1.5-mile hike.

Nearby Attractions

You're not far from John Mahon Nature Park (Hike 5) and the UF Cultural Complex, home to the UF NATL Nature Trails (Hike 18) and the Florida Museum of Natural History: **flmnh.ufl.edu.** The University of Florida is just up the street and offers tours of its historic campus: **ufl.edu/visitors.** Grab great eats nearby at another Gainesville institution, Burrito Brothers Taco Co.: **burritobros.com.**

Directions

From I-75, Exit 387, Newberry Road, drive east 2.8 miles past the Oaks Mall and continue toward the University of Florida. The road becomes University Boulevard after it passes John Mahon Nature Park (Hike 5). At the intersection of NW 34th Street (CR 121), turn left. The right turn onto 5th Avenue comes up very quickly, with a tiny sign hidden between residences. The good news is there is no charge for parking. However, there are only three parking spaces. Alternate parking is possible farther up NW 34th Street at a city park on the right, connecting to this entrance via a sidewalk. Parking is also available at another entrance to the park off 8th Avenue on NW 31st Drive.

7 Longleaf Flatwoods Reserve

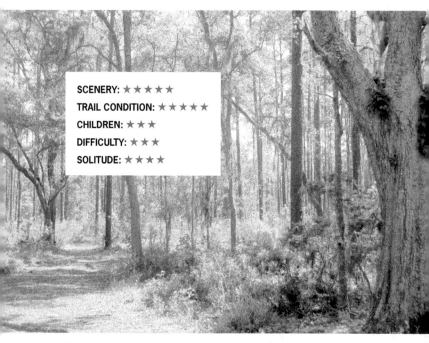

SCENERY: ★ ★ ★ ★ ★
TRAIL CONDITION: ★ ★ ★ ★ ★
CHILDREN: ★ ★ ★
DIFFICULTY: ★ ★ ★
SOLITUDE: ★ ★ ★ ★

FOLLOWING THE TRAIL THROUGH SANDHILL HABITAT

GPS TRAILHEAD COORDINATES: N29° 33.914' W82° 11.354'

DISTANCE & CONFIGURATION: 4.4-mile loop

HIKING TIME: 2 hours

HIGHLIGHTS: Healthy sandhill habitat, pine savanna, cypress dome

ACCESS: Daily, sunrise–sunset. Free.

MAPS: USGS *Rochelle,* at trailhead kiosk

FACILITIES: Primitive group camping area

WHEELCHAIR ACCESS: None

COMMENTS: Pets welcome. Trails are shared with equestrians and cyclists.

CONTACTS: St. Johns Water Management District: 386-329-4404; **sjrwmd.com.**; Alachua County Environmental Protection Department, Land Conservation Division: 352-264-6800; **alachuacounty.us.**

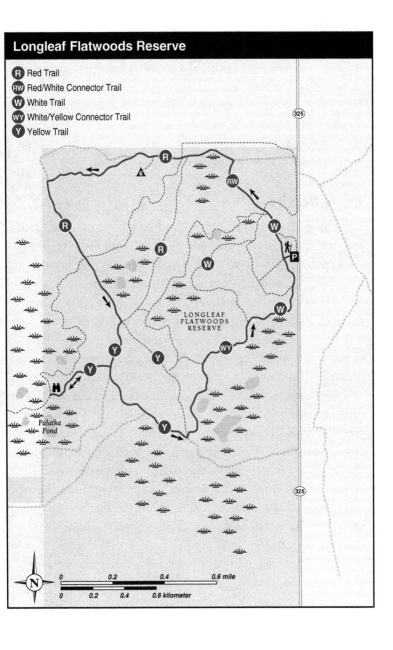

Longleaf Flatwoods Reserve

- **R** Red Trail
- **RW** Red/White Connector Trail
- **W** White Trail
- **WY** White/Yellow Connector Trail
- **Y** Yellow Trail

LONGLEAF
FLATWOODS
RESERVE

*Palatka
Pond*

| 0 | 0.2 | 0.4 | 0.6 mile |

| 0 | 0.2 | 0.4 | 0.6 kilometer |

Overview

North of Cross Creek and Micanopy, this St. Johns Water Management District property has a multiloop trail system through a variety of habitats across 2,850 acres of upland watershed between Orange Lake, Lake Lochloosa, and Paynes Prairie. The trails were built for and are shared by equestrians, as they are blazed with diamond markers along forest roads; however, they are interesting and firm enough underfoot that this is a worthwhile hiking destination.

Route Details

From the gate, walk up a short entrance trail to the trailhead kiosk and pick up a trail map. This hike follows the perimeter of all the loops, starting with the White Trail. Turn right and walk north into an open landscape of pine savanna, with scattered longleaf pines rising from a saw palmetto understory. In spring, wooly pawpaw bloom along the edges of the trail, rising out of a bed of bracken fern.

As the trail comes up to a wall of vegetation, a firebreak joins in from the right and the trail turns left. After a quarter mile you reach the junction of the White Trail with the Red/White Connector Trail. This intersection is a little confusing. Turn to the left, and as you see the white blazes lead off to the south—the White Trail is the shortest of the loops in the preserve—turn right to follow the red blazes to continue along the perimeter trail. You walk into a broad, open landscape of young pines that seems like it's under restoration, as the longleaf pines here are much younger, excepting some tall, skinny, spindly ones that stand out sharply against the sky. There is little shade. The footpath can get damp. Clusters of wild bachelor's button rise from the sand.

At 0.5 mile the trail makes a wide swing to the right away from a treeline. If the shiny lyonia is in bloom, it will be laden with bright fuchsia-colored blossoms. Reaching a graded road at a T intersection, the Red/White Connector Trail turns left to follow the road. The limerock road curves through a bayhead, heading for the sandhills. A double red blaze marks the beginning of the Red Trail loop. Continue straight ahead, passing a campsite symbol. The path narrows, entering puddles of shade cast by post oaks, blackjack oaks, and turkey oaks. All decked out in resurrection fern, the live oaks here are of significant size. Passing the turnoff for the group campsite at 0.9 mile, you continue straight ahead through the shade. Pine duff underfoot makes the walking easy.

As you see more pines throughout the forest, the landscape dips into swales in various directions, looking like they're tracing the path of an underground stream. Some of the pines have catfaces—deep, tall cuts in their trunks—from turpentine tapping, some with the old metal flashing still embedded in the tree. To the left, longleaf pine and wiregrass go on as far as you can see through the open understory. The trail reaches a T intersection with a forest road coming in from the right and makes a left, turning south to follow the road. You briefly see the property fence off to the right. Pinewoods milkweed splays across the wiregrass, showing off its pale

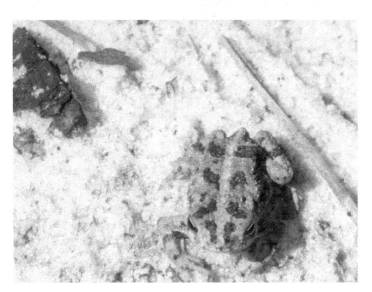

OAK TOAD AT PALATKA POND

pink flowers in spring. A transition zone comes at 1.6 miles, where the tall pines start, and you enter a scrub habitat for a brief stretch. You reach the junction of the Red and Yellow Trails at 2 miles. This is the bottom of the Red Loop. Turn right to stay on the perimeter trail, heading south.

On this part of the trail, the habitat to your left doesn't look as healthy as the ones you've walked through. It's more like an old pasture that has grown back up with opportunistic trees, like laurel oaks, along its perimeter. At the junction of yellow blazes and yellow blazes, turn right. The trail descends into a shady upland forest with a mix of pines among the oaks. The tall columnar tree trunks ahead make up a cypress dome, complete with frogs croaking in the marsh that surrounds it. The trail faces it briefly before it curves to the left. This spur trail leads you deeper into the shady forest before emerging at a spot with bright white sand and pond cypress trees on the rim of the pine forest. Although there is no sign here to confirm it, this seems to be the location of Palatka Pond on the preserve map, and the pond is dry or has retreated well back into the open prairie in front of you. The blazes simply end here.

Turn around and follow the yellow blazes back to the main perimeter trail, reaching it at 2.8 miles. Turn right. The trail comes to a fork almost immediately; keep to the left. It leads you out into former pastureland, an open, sunny area where tall grasses dominate. Young longleaf has been planted to restart a forest. As you come to an intersection with an unmarked graded forest road at 3 miles, continue straight ahead. The landscape drops off to the right, indicating the potential of a wetland area amid the prairie grasses. The trail turns to the north. The forest is sandhills but relatively open. You see a line of pines off to the right. Passing a double diamond marker, the trail reaches another confusing junction, this one with double yellow on two sides of a post and no blazes straight ahead. Make a sharp left at this post, and then an immediate sharp right at the fork to stay on the Yellow Loop. The trail now follows the ecotone between upland forest and former pasture.

At the junction of white and yellow blazes, turn right to follow the White/Yellow Connector Trail. It leads you into well-established wet pine flatwoods where low spots collect water after a rain. Following the white blazes past sweetgum trees and a skinny pine bent over like a catapult, step over a swale where water drains across the footpath. Reaching a Y junction with the bottom of the White Loop at 3.9 miles, turn right to finish the last segment. Tall pines provide shade. The forest on the right is dense, with loblolly bay in the background, grapevines draped over shiny lyonia, and the crooked forms of rusty lyonia reaching out toward the trail from a thicket of saw palmetto. As the trail curves through the shade of a small oak hammock, the road is to your right. Emerging along the edge of a grassy pine savanna, you can see the sparkle of sunlight off the metal roof of the kiosk in the distance. You reach the kiosk at 4.3 miles. Turn right to exit to the parking area, wrapping up a 4.4-mile hike.

Nearby Attractions

Marjorie Kinnan Rawlings lived and wrote her best-known novels at Cross Creek: **floridastateparks.org/marjoriekinnanrawlings.** The Yearling Restaurant is known far and wide for its distinctive Cracker cuisine (native Florida cuisine based on old-time recipes): **yearling restaurant.net.** In Evinston, Wood & Swink General Store, built in 1882, contains Florida's oldest post office: **facebook.com/pages /The-Wood-and-Swink-Preservation-Society/168124363234947.**

Directions

From I-75, Exit 374, Micanopy, drive east on CR 234 toward US 441. Turn south on US 441 and continue through Micanopy, passing the blinker, to make the left onto CR 346 after 1.5 miles. Drive 5.1 miles northeast on CR 346. When it ends at CR 325, turn left. Continue 2.6 miles north to the large parking area on the left.

Mill Creek Preserve

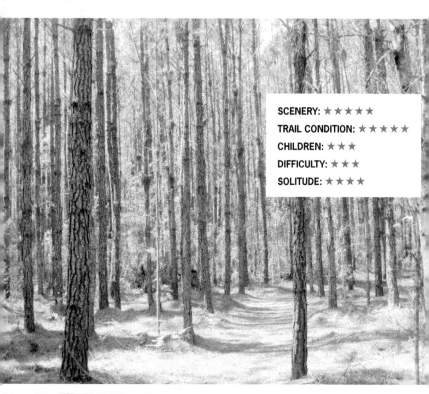

SCENERY: ★ ★ ★ ★ ★
TRAIL CONDITION: ★ ★ ★ ★ ★
CHILDREN: ★ ★
DIFFICULTY: ★ ★
SOLITUDE: ★ ★ ★ ★

PINE PLANTATION AT MILL CREEK PRESERVE

GPS TRAILHEAD COORDINATES: N29° 52.767' W82° 29.828'
DISTANCE & CONFIGURATION: 4.8-mile double balloon
HIKING TIME: 2.25 hours
HIGHLIGHTS: Big trees, waterfall, ravines, historic road
ACCESS: Daily, sunrise–sunset. Free.
MAPS: USGS *Worthington Springs*, at trailhead kiosk
FACILITIES: Trailhead kiosk, benches along the trails
WHEELCHAIR ACCESS: None
COMMENTS: Pets welcome. Trails are open to cyclists.
CONTACTS: Alachua County Environmental Protection Department, Land Conservation Division: 352-264-6800; **alachuacounty.us**

Mill Creek Preserve

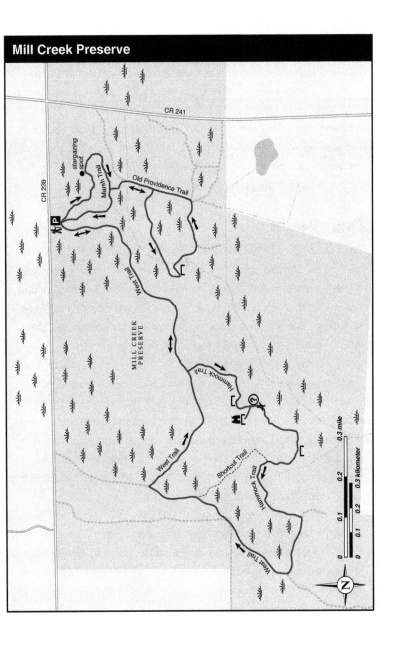

Overview

North of Alachua, Mill Creek Preserve, part of the Alachua County Forever program, encompasses more than 1,200 acres of unexpected finds, including a historic road and a waterfall 5 feet tall. Magnificent spruce pines and swamp chestnut oaks tower over a deeply folded landscape that drains in every direction, its rugged slopes home to the southernmost American beech forest in the United States. A screen of pine plantation hides these finds from passersby, so you have to hike into the preserve to discover its treasures.

Route Details

From the trailhead kiosk, two trails, the West Trail and the Marsh Trail, lead off in different directions. You can hike one or both; our route covers both, starting with the yellow-blazed West Trail. Turn right and follow the fence to the West Trail, which leads you down an old forest road through a pine plantation. The surroundings are a little boring, but it's worth the walk to get to the heart of the preserve.

Reaching a T intersection, turn right. Other plants grow among the planted pines, trying to take back their habitat from this man-made landscape. Ferns rise out of a jumble of rusting farm equipment. The poles along the trail mark gopher tortoise burrows. You emerge into a large clearing with a squiggly trail sign. Continue straight, following the yellow blazes into the next pine plantation. Past a couple of unmarked side trails, you see what looks like a depression marsh beyond the trees to the left.

At 0.6 mile a large log bench and sign call your attention to the beginning of the orange-blazed Hammock Trail. Turn left. Narrowing to a footpath, the trail drops gently downhill. Spruce pines tower overhead as the trail passes its first American beech. Its leaves are large and oval, with sawtooth edges. Beneath the tree you'll find beechnuts, a foraging food for squirrels, foxes, and raccoons. As beeches are a deciduous tree, the best time to visit is in spring, when new leaves are on the trees.

After crossing a plank bridge over a little stream, you see many more interpretive signs and labels on plants and trees, such as sparkleberry, saw palmetto, and loblolly pine. At a sign that points to the right, follow the side path along a winding creek and beneath an enormous swamp chestnut oak to where it ends at a bench overlooking the creek. You've hiked a mile.

Back at the main trail is a kiosk explaining the American beech and the importance of this southernmost beech forest. Several excellent specimens of the tree are just past the sign. The trail drops down to cross the creek on a nicely designed open-grate footbridge made of recycled metal, a work of art with a butterfly motif. Scrambling uphill, you see more beech trees, water oaks, musclewoods, and even a Florida sugar maple. Identification markers help greatly in teaching you the trees and plants of this forest.

As you move away from the waterways, there is an obvious transition in the understory. Just beyond an interpretive sign for highbush blueberry, near a bench made out of a log, there is a bluff oak ringed with woodpecker holes. The landscape rolls downhill to the left into a depression. At 1.3 miles you reach the junction with the Shortcut Trail at a bench and kiosk. Skipping the Shortcut Trail for the longer Hammock Trail, you'll find more identified plants. An oak that has fallen over has sprouted its limbs into small trees. As the trail meanders between tall trees, planted slash pines begin to invade the forest.

By 1.6 miles the Hammock Trail ends at the West Trail. Turn right. You're back on a forest road, following the yellow blazes. The open area looks suspiciously like the one near the beginning of the hike with the gopher tortoise burrows, but don't be fooled; it's not. Unmarked trails go off in all directions. Follow the yellow wiggly arrow sign (and parking symbol) to stay on the correct path. Beyond the corner post of a fence, the yellow blazes stay to the right, with an open scrubby flatwoods area to the left. At 2.1 miles the lime-green–blazed Shortcut Trail comes in from the right. Continue straight. The West Trail makes a broad swath between scrubby flatwoods and pine forest. Once you can see power lines and passing traffic in the distance, the trail turns left at a yellow marker with a parking symbol on it, back into the woods as a forest road.

Horse sugar, or sweetleaf—with leaves that look a little like a small rhododendron—grows in a small clearing where we watched several woodpeckers in the trees, including a pileated woodpecker and a downy woodpecker. An abandoned road leads to the left. There are tall trees all around, including spruce pine and loblolly pine. The shady path drops downhill, completing the loop with the Hammock Trail at 2.6 miles. Continue straight ahead on the West Trail, passing through the clearing with the gopher tortoise burrows. Make a left at the next trail junction to head back out to the parking area.

Reaching the kiosk at the parking area after 3.3 miles, make a right to start the Marsh Trail. The blue blazes lead you behind an interpretive display to a Y intersection. Keep left. Unlike the West Trail, this is a footpath carved out of the pine plantation. Gallberry thrives beneath the slash pines. A side trail leads to an observation spot along a small marshy prairie in the pines, with a canted bench that looks up to the sky.

At 3.7 miles you reach the trail junction with the white-blazed Old Providence Trail. Turn left down a short connector trail, and left again. You cross a culvert and face a long, straight forest road. This is a portion of the Old Providence Road, once connecting Fort Call, established during the Second Seminole War in 1845 near Worthington Springs, with Newnansville, the seat of Alachua County from 1828 until 1853, now a ghost town. Keep alert because you only walk down this path briefly before the trail makes an abrupt right.

On this path, the habitat transitions to bluff forest, where shiny lyonia grows beneath Southern magnolia. At a grassy spot with a marker that points left, you enter deep shade along Townsend Creek. If the creek is running—depending on recent rains and overall drought—you'll see a waterfall dropping 5 feet over an overhang in the narrow ravine created by the creek. Benches let you sit and watch the water. As the trail climbs, towering trees create a high canopy. The undulating landscape is thanks to feeder streams that pump water into the creek after a rain.

By 4.2 miles the trail widens, with lush bottomland forest downhill to the right. After passing a small clearing, the trail climbs up a straightaway, emerging into a large clearing with trails leading in multiple directions. Turn left and you're back on the Old Providence Road, following the white blazes. Completing the loop by 4.5 miles, continue straight ahead. After the culvert, turn right on the connector back to the Marsh Trail. At the T intersection, turn left.

The blue-blazed Marsh Trail continues its loop through the pine plantation. A tiny clearing on the left shows off a relict patch of the original scrubby flatwoods that the planted pines obliterated. Curving right, the trail heads straight down a corridor flanked by slash pines. Making a sharp right past another little clearing, you can see the kiosk ahead. You complete this loop after 4.8 miles, emerging at the kiosk and parking area.

Nearby Attractions

Florida's largest live oak tree is at Cellon Oak Park, with a trunk more than 30 feet in diameter: **alachuacounty.us.** Historic Alachua has many places to dine; our favorite is Conestoga's Restaurant for a hearty steak or burger: **conestogasrestaurant.com.** One of Florida's top art and antiques destinations, High Springs is a launch point for outdoor adventures on the Santa Fe River: **visitgainesville.com /nearby-towns/high-springs.**

Directions

From I-75, Exit 399, High Springs/Alachua, drive south on US 441 to the traffic light with CR 235, one block past Main Street. Turn north. Veer left onto CR 241. Continue 5 miles to its intersection with CR 239. Turn left. Drive another third of a mile to the preserve entrance on the left.

9

Morningside Nature Center

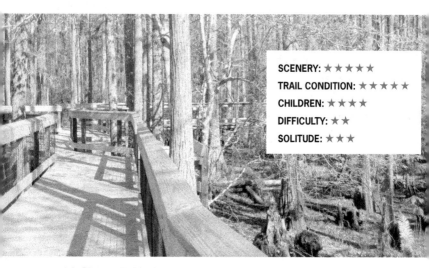

BOARDWALK THROUGH A CYPRESS DOME

GPS TRAILHEAD COORDINATES: N29° 39.346' W82° 16.608'

DISTANCE & CONFIGURATION: 4.6-mile loop

HIKING TIME: 2.75 hours

HIGHLIGHTS: Scenic, hilly terrain above Hogtown Creek; ancient trees; spring wildflowers

ACCESS: Daily, 8 a.m.–6 p.m.; farm open Tuesday–Saturday, 9 a.m.–4:30 p.m. Free.

MAPS: USGS *Gainesville East*, on trailhead kiosk

FACILITIES: Restrooms and water fountain at nature center and at the picnic area, benches along the trail, Living History Farm, replica American Indian village, bird blind

WHEELCHAIR ACCESS: Limited to nature center area; with some minimal assistance, can include Cypress Dome Boardwalk behind the nature center

COMMENTS: Pets not permitted. Reenactors from the Friends of Nature Parks re-create pioneer life on Saturdays September–May in the Living History Farm and lead wildflower walks in fall. Two annual events—the Cane Boil, held in late November, and the Farm and Forest Festival, held in April—draw thousands of visitors for the day. Check before visiting, as the park may be closed for short periods during prescribed burns.

CONTACTS: Morningside Nature Center: 352-334-3326. City of Gainesville Department of Parks, Recreation and Cultural Affairs, Nature Operations Division: 352-334-5067; **natureoperations.org; facebook.com/cityofgainesvillenature**. Friends of Nature Parks: **friendsofnatureparks.org**.

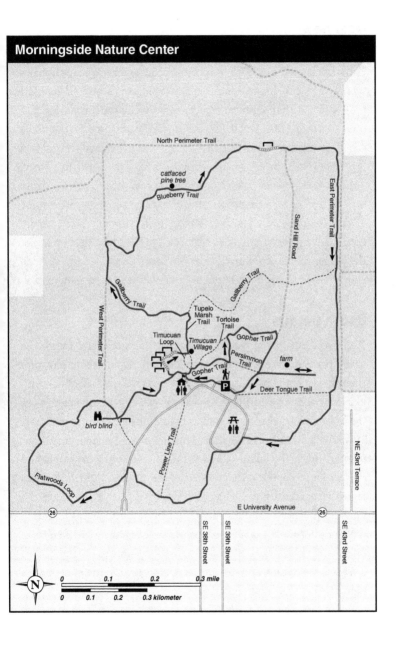

Morningside Nature Center

Overview

The City of Gainesville's flagship nature park, Morningside Nature Center, opened in 1970. Protecting 268 acres of natural habitats within city limits—including a significant stand of longleaf pine savanna that survived thanks to its value for turpentine tapping between 1909 and 1948—the park hosts some of the area's most-attended outdoor festivals. It is a major regional destination for school and church groups because of its Living History Farm, a 10-acre re-created family farm where historical buildings from around the region were brought together to depict pioneer life in the 1870s. The park includes an extensive, well-maintained trail system with many options for long and short loops. This hike follows one of the longer routes, keeping close to the park's perimeter, but you can shorten it or change it up based on what you see on the park map.

Route Details

Walk west out of the parking area, past the kiosk, and follow the paved path to the environmental education center, where a map of the trail system is posted. Though the center is normally busy with local school groups during the week, you can stop in the foyer to use the restrooms and pick up a map before heading out on the trail. Turn right. At the CYPRESS DOME BOARDWALK sign, turn right to enjoy this broad boardwalk snaking between the cypress trees and the marsh ferns below them. Benches are inset at numerous spots along the boardwalk, providing places to watch lizards race across the railings. The end of the boardwalk guides you into a small clearing with an interpretive area for educators to share the clash of cultures between Spanish explorers and the native Timucua in the 1500s. Turn left and walk away from the environmental center, entering the pine flatwoods on a nice broad path.

By 0.4 mile you reach a T intersection with the Gallberry Trail, blazed with yellow triangles. Turn left. Yellow-eyed grass blooms in the footpath, and the shiny blueberries sparkle with white blooms in early spring. Even though this preserve is inside the city limits of Gainesville, the forest is managed with prescribed burns, so expect to see char marks on the pines. The Gallberry Trail meets the Perimeter Trail at a T intersection. Turn right to follow the blue blazes. Keep alert for a trail going to the right amid a mound of grapevines at a half-hidden post with double yellow diamonds. Turn right to follow the Blueberry Trail through a boggy spot, where the footpath is slightly squishy and bog wildflowers, such as small butterwort, star-rush, and wild bachelor's button, thrive. As the trail climbs, longleaf pines tower overhead. The understory is very open; you can see a great distance in every direction, providing the illusion of not being in a city.

At 1.2 miles the Blueberry Trail reaches a T intersection with the North Perimeter Trail. Turn right, reaching a boardwalk through a cypress dome, with a view of the marsh in the center of the dome. Pass the junction with Sandhill Road. As the trail gains a little elevation, the habitat shifts, with sand live oaks and turkey oaks overhead and young longleaf pines clustered together in the open understory. Curving to stay within the property boundary, the trail faces a vista filled with colorful wildflowers each fall. You come to a junction with the Gallberry Trail, where young longleaf pines are accented by the haze of soft grasses beneath them. Stay left to continue along the Perimeter Trail.

A fence towers next to the trail. It was a necessary addition around the Living History Farm, to secure the historical buildings and to keep deer out of the gardens, but it does detract from the beauty of this part of the walk. Reaching the next intersection at 2 miles, the trail to the right is a shortcut—it follows the fence back to the parking area where you started. Stay to the left. The Perimeter Trail curves right to avoid a bayhead swamp. At a T intersection with an old house, the blue blazes lead you left. After the next sharp right, the trail continues down a long straightaway under the pines. You see picnic tables ahead in the picnic area not far from the parking area; it has restrooms and a water fountain.

Leaving the picnic area, the trail isn't obvious but it follows the edge of the parking area to the south. The blue blazes lead you down the Ecotone Trail. Turning right sharply, the trail parallels FL 26 as it burrows through a thicket of gallberry under the pines, the traffic noise a counterpoint to the quiet immersion in longleaf pine habitat you enjoyed earlier. At 2.5 miles the Power Line Trail joins in from the right. A few minutes later, you reach the park road. Turn left and walk down the road a short distance to find the entrance to the Flatwoods Loop Trail; just before the park gate, look for the blue blaze on the right-hand side.

Quickly narrowing down to a tight corridor, the trail enters pine flatwoods. Catbrier drapes over understory plants, and pine needles dangle from everything. The pines above are very tall. Beneath the red maples, you find a bench. At 3.2 miles turn right onto the Bird Blind Trail and walk down it a short ways to a four-way junction. The bird blind is to the right. It's a wooden structure like a small shed; you sit inside it on a bench, peering out of a tiny slit in the wood, a bird identification book handy. The bird feeders attract songbirds, particularly titmice. From the blind, walk back up to the four-way intersection and continue straight ahead, following the trail as it winds through the pine flatwoods. Passing the entrance to the Cypress Dome Boardwalk, you've completed a loop.

While it's quicker to walk back past your car to get to the Living History Farm, the trail network will get you there on paths that you haven't explored yet. Pass by the front of the nature center and its native plant garden, and walk around the back side. Look for the pink blazes of the Persimmon Trail to your right. At a Y intersection, keep left. The trail leads you into the sandhills. Passing a trail to the right, the path makes a left turn and you find a confirmation pink blaze that looks like lichen on a tree. At the T intersection, turn right, reaching the Gopher Trail at 3.8 miles. It, too, follows an ecotone between pine flatwoods and sandhills.

At the next intersection, you see the perimeter fence of the farm again. Turn right onto Sandhill Road. By 4 miles you are at the entrance gate to the Living History Farm. Open until 4:30 p.m., it has several buildings, including a historical schoolhouse, farmhouse, and blacksmith shop, in a large clearing in the pine forest. An orange grove grows near the pioneer school, and a dairy cow grazes in the barnyard. After a wander through the farm, which takes about a quarter mile to walk around, exit at the gate and walk down the broad path to the parking area. Returning to the kiosk, you've completed a 4.6-mile circuit of Morningside Nature Center.

Nearby Attractions

Along Newnans Lake—where a collection of dugout canoes more than 7,000 years old were discovered during low water levels in 2000—walk sometimes soggy trails into an ancient cypress floodplain: **sjrwmd.com/recreationguide/newnanslake.** Pretty Palm Point Park provides a panorama of the cypress-lined lakeshore from beneath ancient live oaks: **natureoperations.org.**

Directions

From I-75, Exit 382, drive east on SE Williston Road (FL 331) for 5.5 miles, crossing US 441 and passing the turnoffs for Main Street (Bivens Arm Nature Park, Hike 3) and SE Fourth Street (to Sweetwater Preserve, Hike 16, and Paynes Prairie Preserve State Park: La Chua Trail, Hike 10). When you reach East University Avenue (FL 20/26), turn right. Keep left where FL 20 and FL 26 diverge to stay on FL 26. Drive 2.2 miles east to the entrance for Morningside Nature Center on the left. Follow the park road to the interior of the preserve to a visitor parking area on the left that adjoins the trailhead kiosk and access to the Living History Farm.

10

Paynes Prairie Preserve State Park:

La Chua Trail

SCENERY: ★ ★ ★ ★ ★
TRAIL CONDITION: ★ ★ ★ ★ ★
CHILDREN: ★ ★
DIFFICULTY: ★
SOLITUDE: ★

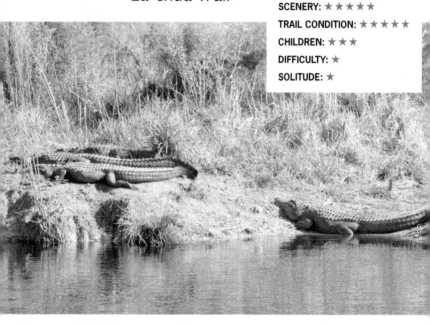

ALLIGATORS SUNNING ALONG THE LA CHUA TRAIL

GPS TRAILHEAD COORDINATES: N29° 36.604' W82° 18.262'

DISTANCE & CONFIGURATION: 3.2-mile out-and-back

HIKING TIME: 1.5 hours

HIGHLIGHTS: Best place to see alligators in the wild in Florida, great birding

ACCESS: Daily, 8 a.m. to one hour before sunset. Entrance fee: $2 per person.

MAPS: USGS *Micanopy,* on trailhead kiosk

FACILITIES: Trailhead kiosk, restroom, benches, observation platforms

WHEELCHAIR ACCESS: 1-mile round-trip on pavement and boardwalk with
great wildlife viewing

COMMENTS: Pets prohibited. If you bring children, keep them close at hand. Do *not*
approach the alligators. Although they look sluggish, they can move very quickly when
they want to.

CONTACTS: Paynes Prairie Preserve State Park: 352-466-3397; **floridastateparks.org
/paynesprairie**

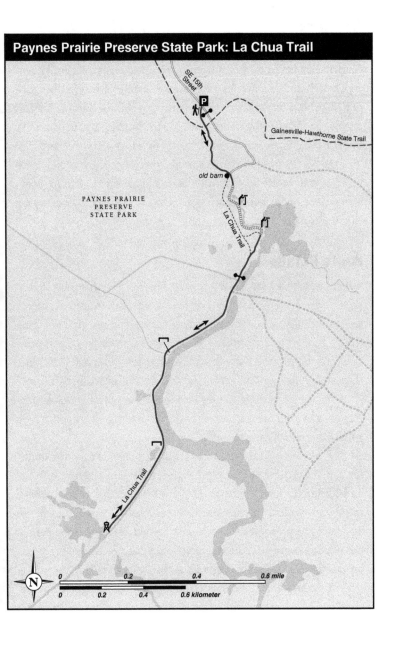

Paynes Prairie Preserve State Park: La Chua Trail

Overview

There's no doubt about it: the place to see gators is the home of the Gators. Not far from the campus of the University of Florida, the La Chua Trail at Paynes Prairie Preserve State Park offers a picture-perfect view of crowds of alligators gathering at the lowest spot in the prairie, where all of the water from the surrounding 188-square-mile watershed ends up. Home to Alachua Sink, where the water vanishes into the Floridan Aquifer, this combination of boardwalk and levee trail lets you choose how far into the wild you want to go to see wildlife up close, with observation decks above the sinks and an observation tower more than a mile out into the prairie itself.

Route Details

Adjoining a kiosk that shows you where to find all of the trails in this state park, the La Chua Trail begins as a sidewalk from the parking area. Winding past a sprawling live oak covered in resurrection fern, the trail comes to a junction with the paved Gainesville–Hawthorne Trail, the same trail you use to visit Sweetwater Preserve (Hike 16) to the north. A pay station, bench, water fountain, and composting toilet mark the entrance to Paynes Prairie Preserve State Park. Neither bicycles nor pets are permitted along the trail past this point, and you'll discover why as you walk along.

Plum trees dot the hillside, with showy blooms in winter drawing your attention away from the high-tension wires overhead. Walk under the crumbling remains of a historic railroad trestle, where cattle once walked through onto Paynes Prairie. Passing enormous live oaks, the path goes through a barn—where interpretive panels talk about five centuries of ranching on the prairie—and out into the open range. The sidewalk meets a boardwalk at 0.3 mile.

This broad boardwalk is one of Gainesville's biggest natural attractions, circling around a site to which visitors have flocked for several centuries, the Alachua Sink. Water flows from all over the surrounding watershed to feed the deep sinkhole that is now in front of you, a karst window into the Floridan Aquifer. Now and then, the sinkhole clogs up, turning Paynes Prairie into an enormous lake. We've seen it happen as recently as the last decade. Most of the time, however, water flows down into it and disappears, never to return to the prairie. At times of very low water, you may see a waterfall falling into the sinkhole's throat.

The boardwalk gently curves around the sink to show it off from several angles, with an observation deck near the end of a natural sluiceway. This waterway connects the upper lake with the lower sinkhole. Wading birds, especially great blue herons and Louisiana herons, will stand along the rushing waters to pluck out their meals. You start seeing the alligators along this stretch. They crawl up the banks of the waterway and sun themselves on the slopes. As you draw closer to a covered observation deck with benches at a half mile, you reach the upper lake, with its rock formation on the far shore. When the prairie was a lake in the late 1800s, steamboats would dock near these rocks, which are shown on old Florida postcards.

Take a close look at the waters below. Those dark specks are alligators, lots of alligators. Depending on the air temperature, there may be more floating in the water than on the banks of the lake. Paynes Prairie has a massive alligator population, and in times of drought, they all seem to end up here. We've seen more alligators along this trail than any other trail in Florida. Keep that in mind as you step off the boardwalk and continue along the trail on the levee. While this is a wonderful trail for wildlife sightings—especially enormous alligators in their natural setting—it's also a place where you need to stay very alert.

The grassy path follows the top of the bluff to the edge of the lake, where another natural sluiceway feeds the prairie's water downhill. You might see rapids, depending on the water level, with alligators lying in wait for stunned fish or other creatures tumbling down the waterway. You'll see gator slides and gator trails right up these banks. There is no fence, nothing to keep you and the alligators apart except your common sense. This is why pets aren't allowed, and why small children shouldn't ramble along on their own.

The channel on the left is a drainage canal built by the ranchers to drain the marshes for their cattle to graze. It pours into the sluice-way through a culvert under the trail. Beyond this gate and culvert, the trail is atop a levee for the remainder of the trek. Alligators commonly gather in the shallows to the left, throwing their massive bodies across the open ground on the far shore. You'll see younger ones floating in the thick vegetation. Don't even think of walking down toward the water's edge.

As you walk along the levee, the waterway on the left becomes shallower. At times, there may be mudflats along it, attracting roseate spoonbills, a colorful pink wading bird we've seen here in the summer months. No matter the time of year, there is always a parade of

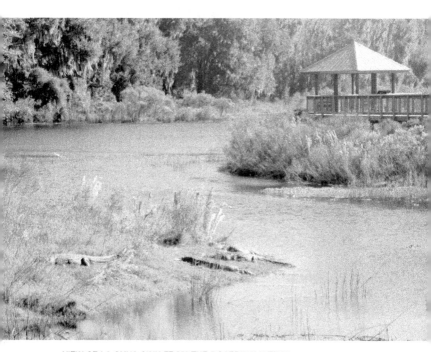

VIEW OF LA CHUA SINK FROM THE BOARDWALK TRAIL

birds, especially in the early morning hours. At 1 mile you reach a bench overlooking the waterway. The trail makes a sharp left here to continue on the levee between the waterway and the marshes.

Open water traces a sinuous curve through the aquatic plants for a while, and then becomes a solid sea of floating greenery. On the right is a lance-leaved arrowhead and water lettuce pool surrounded by tall grasses. Looking off to both horizons, you can see how Paynes Prairie is a bowl surrounded by bluffs, and you're in the thick of it. The next bench is a quarter mile later. Sitting here, you can see alligators lazing on dry ground along the marsh.

A patchwork of water and aquatic grasses shimmers in the sun as you continue along the levee, just above the level of the waters. Since this trail remains busy, it's unlikely you'll come across alligators sunning on it, but if you do, don't even try to pass them to continue down the trail. If they don't move on your approach, that's not a good thing—it means they aren't afraid of people. Back off. While they look sluggish, alligators can run fast enough in spurts to take down a deer.

You reach the observation tower at the end of the La Chua Trail after 1.6 miles. While it's only one flight up—the Wacahoota Trail (Hike 11) on the south rim has the five-story tower—it provides an excellent perch for surveying this flat mosaic of marshes, deeper to the east, shallower to the west. On a clear day, you can look back to the treeline and see the entire mile of open landscape that you just traversed. Beyond the bounty of wildlife, the most interesting part of Paynes Prairie is the colors and patterns and textures of the marsh.

Leaving the observation tower, return the way you came. At 1.9 miles the trail curves past the bench along a patch of open water, where alligators gather along every available stretch of dry bluff on sunny days. Passing the second bench at 2.2 miles, the trail continues to parallel the broad waterway. A gate on the right, which leads to another levee, is padlocked. Good thing, as a big gator slide goes up and over that levee. Back through the main gate, over the culvert, you're on the bluffs again along the sluiceway. From this angle, you might see the alligators at the base of the near bluff more easily.

At 2.7 miles you return to the boardwalk. Follow it back around Alachua Sink, taking one more opportunity to spot alligators in the lake and along the shoreline. A water fountain is right near a bench by the barn as you leave the boardwalk. Continue back through the barn, under the trestle, and across the Gainesville–Hawthorne Trail, returning to the parking area after 3.2 miles.

Nearby Attractions

As you can see at the trailhead kiosk, there are a lot of trails at Paynes Prairie. This is the only one on the north rim. The Wacahoota Trail (Hike 11) makes a good gateway for the south rim trails. Sweetwater Preserve (Hike 16) is just north along SE 15th Street. On this side of Gainesville, you're closest to the Southeast Historic Bed & Breakfast District: **facebook.com/pages /Gainesvilles-SE-Historic-Bed-Breakfast-District/294431106660.**

Directions

From I-75, Exit 382, drive east on SE Williston Road (FL 331), crossing US 441 after 4.3 miles. Continue around the curve past the western entrance to the preserve and the traffic light. Turn right onto SE Fourth Street, which curves slightly to become SE 21st Avenue. Turn right on SE 15th Street. Continue past Bouleware Springs Park (with access to Hike 16) to the park entrance at a sharp left curve in the road next to a subdivision. Go straight ahead on Camp Ranch Road to enter the parking area down a short drive under the oak canopy.

11

Paynes Prairie
Preserve State Park:
Wacahoota Trail

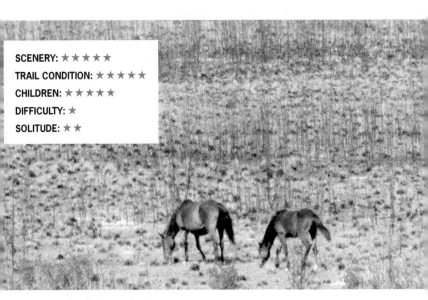

SCENERY: ★ ★ ★ ★ ★
TRAIL CONDITION: ★ ★ ★ ★ ★
CHILDREN: ★ ★ ★ ★
DIFFICULTY: ★
SOLITUDE: ★ ★

WILD HORSES GRAZING ON PAYNES PRAIRIE

GPS TRAILHEAD COORDINATES: N29° 32.848' W82° 17.640'

DISTANCE & CONFIGURATION: 1.1-mile balloon

HIKING TIME: 45 minutes

HIGHLIGHTS: Five-story observation tower, visitor center with interpretive information

ACCESS: Daily, 8 a.m.–sunset. Entrance fee: $2 per pedestrian or cyclist; $4 per single-occupant vehicle; $6 per vehicle with up to 8 people.

MAPS: USGS *Micanopy*, available at ranger station

FACILITIES: Trailhead kiosk, restrooms, benches, visitor center, observation platform

WHEELCHAIR ACCESS: Paved path from the parking area to the visitor center and observation tower, where a ramp leads to an observation platform

COMMENTS: Pets are welcome, but not on Cones Dike. Bring your binoculars. You can see herds of wild horses from the tower. The visitor center is open daily, 9 a.m.–4 p.m.

CONTACTS: Paynes Prairie Preserve State Park: 352-466-3397; **floridastateparks.org /paynesprairie**

Paynes Prairie Preserve State Park: Wacahoota Trail

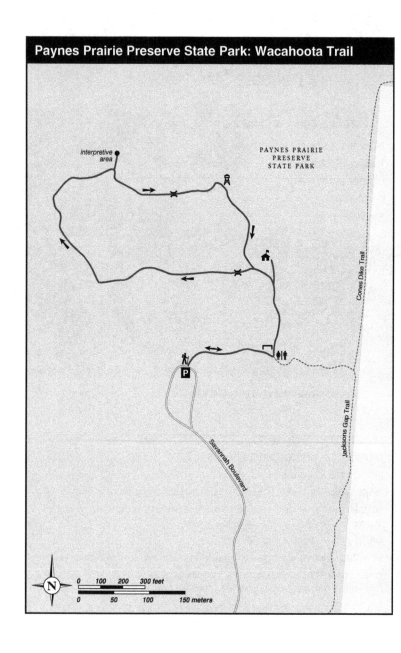

PAYNES PRAIRIE
PRESERVE
STATE PARK

Overview

Established in 1971 and covering more than 21,000 acres, Paynes Prairie Preserve State Park encompasses the vast, shallow limestone basin that botanist William Bartram referred to as the Great Alachua Savannah in 1774. It's a big place to wrap your mind around, which is why we suggest this hike as a launch point to the rest of the preserve. The Wacahoota Trail leads you to the Alachua Savannah Visitor Center, with its interpretive exhibits and films, and to a five-story observation tower that provides the best overview of just how big Paynes Prairie is. Part of the loop is a nature trail with a gentle introduction to the upland habitats above the prairie basin. It also provides access to longer hikes, such as Cones Dike, Jackson Gap, and the Chacala Trail.

Route Details

Start your walk by passing the Birding Trail kiosk, following the sidewalk into the woods. Live oaks provide a well-knit canopy overhead, with hickory and Southern magnolia joining them in the upland forest. You pass a side trail leading to the restrooms and to the Jackson Gap Trail, which connects to the Cones Dike and Chacala Trails. The sidewalk heads downhill, reaching the visitor center. Take some time to visit the exhibits and watch the short film for an introduction to the prairie and its habitats; it's a great help with plant and animal identification along the way. Back on the path, follow it down the slope around the side of the visitor center and you'll see a sign for WACAHOOTA TRAIL. Turn left onto the footpath.

Crossing over a small bridge over an ephemeral tributary flowing toward the prairie, the trail leads into the heart of a hardwood forest along the prairie's rim. Live oaks grow particularly large here, and there are many cabbage palms in the understory. You see sweetgum and hickory scattered throughout. Grapevines dangle in a tangled puzzle from the taller oaks. There is a definite slope to the landscape to the right as the trail turns left and uphill, coming to a broad opening between the trees.

Around a quarter mile, the trail turns right and starts heading downhill, the path softly carpeted by pine needles. A line of slash pines parallels the trail on the left. In the open understory beneath them, you may spy a flock of turkeys browsing. Tall, chunky laurel oaks intermingle through this older forest. The trail drops downhill under the curved limbs of live oaks. Past some limestone boulders—the prairie and its surrounding landscape is karst, home to sinkholes, caves, and springs—there is a large fallen oak on the right providing footholds for fungi.

As the trail descends toward the prairie, you see the flattening of the landscape in the distance, the prairie filling the far horizon glimpsed through a green screen of leaves. Turn right, and the trail follows the prairie's edge, staying in the shade. At a fork in the trail, keep left. This path leads to a small interpretive area with a big salt-making kettle and a closed gate out to the prairie. The fence dates back to the days of cattle ranching on the prairie. You've walked a half mile. Head back up the slope to the main trail, and turn left. Cross a second bridge over the tributary that splashes down through the forest.

Walking under ancient live oaks laden with Spanish moss, you can wonder if these same trees rustled in the breeze as Bartram stood here and took in the beauty of the Great Alachua Savannah in 1774. While dikes and canals altered the prairie in more recent centuries due to cattle ranching, the park's mission is to preserve what Bartram saw, and to that end, you may see free-range Spanish horses and bison from the top of the observation tower. Where the footpath meets the sidewalk, turn left to follow the walkway up and start the five-story climb.

A glider chair lets you sit and enjoy the breeze, or do like most visitors and stand at the railing, scanning the horizon for horses. We've been fortunate to spot the small herd, sometimes with foals, on every one of our visits over the past several years. Across the prairie, Gainesville sits on the bluffs beyond the trees; a few buildings peep out over the trees toward the northwest. The La Chua Trail (Hike 10) is directly north on the north rim; you might be able to make out its smaller observation tower on a clear day. Watch the sky for raptors.

After you descend the tower, turn left. Follow the sidewalk up past the visitor center, keeping right at the fork. You pass another enormous live oak as you finish the loop at the back side of the trail sign at 0.9 mile. Continue up the sidewalk to exit, returning to the parking area after 1.1 miles.

Nearby Attractions

From this same trailhead, you can take a round-trip of up to 8.3 miles on Cones Dike into the heart of the prairie. It's similar to the La Chua Trail (Hike 10) with fewer alligators, fewer hikers, and no observation deck at the end. The 1.3-mile Jackson Gap Trail connects to the Chacala Trail, a 6.2-mile multiuse upland loop shared with equestrians. All of these trails can be cycled. In addition, the Lake Trail (requiring a drive to another trailhead north of the Puc Puggy campground, another feature of this park) provides an easy-to-access spot for birding and reptile-watching from a short boardwalk along Lake Wauberg: **floridastateparks.org/paynesprairie.**

Directions

From I-75, Exit 374, Micanopy, drive east on CR 234 toward US 441. Turn north on US 441 and continue to the park entrance on the right. Once you're inside the park, drive straight down Savannah Boulevard—the beautifully canopied main road through the park—all the way to its end at a parking area adjoining the Great Florida Birding Trail kiosk.

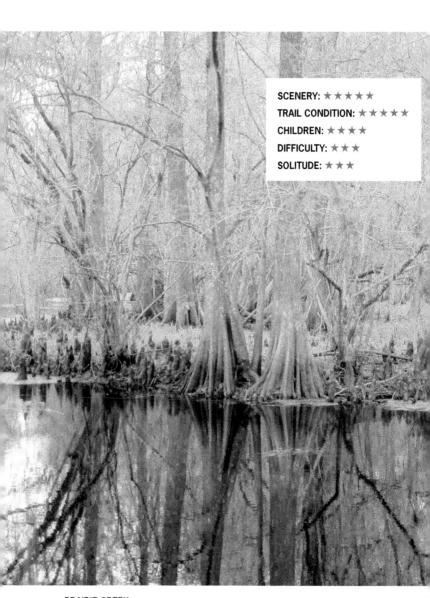

SCENERY: ★ ★ ★ ★ ★
TRAIL CONDITION: ★ ★ ★ ★ ★
CHILDREN: ★ ★ ★
DIFFICULTY: ★ ★
SOLITUDE: ★ ★ ★

PRAIRIE CREEK

GPS TRAILHEAD COORDINATES: N29° 35.773' W82° 13.695'

DISTANCE & CONFIGURATION: 4.7-mile balloon

HIKING TIME: 2.25 hours

HIGHLIGHTS: Ancient trees, vast floodplain forest, views of Prairie Creek

ACCESS: Daily, sunrise–sunset. Free.

MAPS: USGS *Rochelle,* at trailhead kiosk

FACILITIES: Trailhead kiosk, portable toilet 0.25 mile east along the Gainesville–Hawthorne Trail, picnic tables at several spots along the trail

WHEELCHAIR ACCESS: Along the edge of the preserve only, on the Gainesville–Hawthorne Trail

COMMENTS: Pets welcome, but bicycles are not allowed. Trails are shared with equestrians. The orange-blazed Jane Walker Trail leads down to the floodplain of Prairie Creek. Because of the cypress strands and mud, it's a difficult wade if it's flooded; better to return when you can see most of the footpath. Mosquitoes can be fierce in the shady spots.

CONTACTS: Alachua Conservation Trust: 352-373-1078; **alachuaconservationtrust.org.** Gainesville–Hawthorne State Trail: 352-466-3397; **floridastateparks.org/gainesville-hawthorne** (for trailhead).

Overview

Draining Newnans Lake into Paynes Prairie, the expansive Prairie Creek floodplain is a beautiful example of a floodplain forest dominated by cypress strands and ancient trees that don't mind a periodic soaking. Acquired and protected by the nonprofit Alachua Conservation Trust, Prairie Creek Preserve provides one of the wildest places to hike close to the city of Gainesville. Within 360 acres protecting the floodplain of Prairie Creek, the trail system immerses you in an expanse of deep, dark forest unlike any other in the region.

Route Details

There are three entrances to the trail system. This hike starts at the one with the best parking, the Witness Tree Junction Trailhead along the Gainesville–Hawthorne State Trail, where there is a picnic table and a kiosk at the entrance to Prairie Creek Preserve. In spring, you may see wild azalea in bloom at the trailhead. Pick up a map at the kiosk.

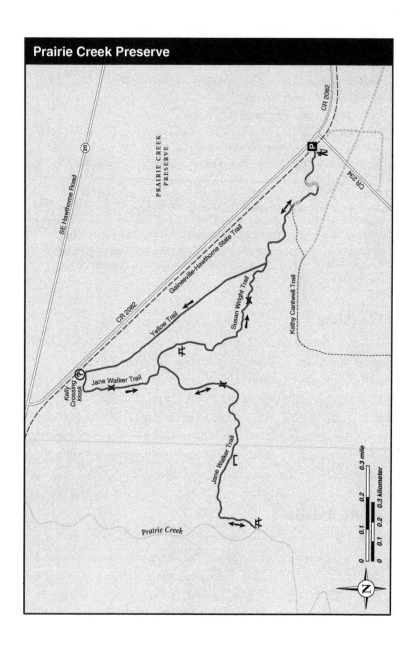

Prairie Creek Preserve

Follow the white blazes into the woods. You soon discover this isn't just the White Trail, but it's also the Wright Trail, dedicated to Susan Wright (who also has a bench honoring her at John Mahon Nature Park, Hike 5). All of the trails in this preserve, each blazed in a different color, honor local conservationists. Starting out in a mix of pine flatwoods and planted slash pines, the trail traverses the lumpy rows left behind in the pine plantation. Birdsong echoes throughout the forest. This pine forest is marshy, with wax myrtle and gallberry in the understory yielding to marsh ferns and tall grasses. Watch your feet, as the footpath gets very rooty.

You reach a substantial boardwalk lifting the trail over the potential flooding from a marsh and cypress strand on the left, which can spill over, nourishing the sphagnum moss below. After the boardwalk ends, the trail plops into a pine plantation, zigzagging between the rows. It's a little higher and drier here, as indicated by the density of bracken fern rising from the pine duff. The forest closes in, creating a canopy of shade. At a T intersection, a sign announces a new boardwalk trail under construction into the cypress dome to the right. Turn left and cross the outflow of this swamp on a long plank-and-log bog bridge, one plank wide, past some rather large cypresses.

After the bridge ends, a sign announces the junction with the Kathy Cantwell Trail, a blue-diamond-blazed trail to the left. Primarily used by equestrians, it's a long, linear connector to the headquarters of the Alachua Conservation Trust. Keep right to stay on the Susan Wright Trail, following the white blazes. It leads into a pine plantation with lots of saw palmetto in the understory. The footpath is damp in places, which lets wild bachelor's button thrive. A cypress strand runs parallel to the right, and the trail stays close to it.

Just after the trail curves between a sink and the cypress swamp, you reach the junction of the Susan Wright Trail with the Yellow Trail at 0.5 mile. Turn right to start the loop. You'll walk through the uplands first, so if there is a need to splash through the floodplain, you'll do that later in the hike. The Yellow Trail follows a mowed, grassy forest road through the pines. Along this straight, broad path, there are mounds of blackberry bushes edged by wax myrtle. At a four-way junction with an unmarked trail, continue straight. A dull thrum of traffic is growing; it echoes through this part of the forest from FL 20, which lies north of the preserve. The canopy closes in overhead.

Passing a large clump of blackberries, you can hear marshland noises to the right, the croaks of frogs and chirps of crickets in the shadows of cypress trees. Entering a hardwood hammock where cabbage palms grow among pines and oaks of significant size, the trail follows a tramway once used for logging. A small depression in the footpath has planks adjoining it for use if water is flowing across the trail. Giant grapevines dangle from the canopy.

As the trail rises out of the swamp, you can see a kiosk in the distance. Passing under power lines, the trail enters another stretch of lush hardwoods. At 1.2 miles you reach Kelly Crossing, the northern trailhead for the preserve, with a picnic bench and kiosk along the Gainesville–Hawthorne State Trail. The Yellow Trail and the orange-blazed Jane Walker Trail meet here. Turn left at the kiosk to follow the orange blazes. If you visit in spring, you may notice the fluffy-looking white blooms of a Florida fringe tree to the right at the base of a large oak.

The Jane Walker Trail has a distinct downhill trend into the floodplain of Prairie Creek as you walk beneath ancient oaks and tall cypresses. The trail makes a 90-degree turn at an orange arrow to stay atop an old dike in the floodplain. Through tall grasses, you walk beneath the power lines again, returning to the swamp forest on the other side. The trail follows a long straightaway. After crossing a small bridge, you see a very large cypress to the right with a sign on its trunk: BOUNDARY, PAYNES PRAIRIE PRESERVE STATE PARK.

By 1.5 miles the tramway ends but the trail continues, meandering through the ancient forest on a clearly defined path. Watch for the junction with the white-blazed Susan Wright Trail. You'll return here after your hike to Prairie Creek. Depending on water levels in Newnans Lake and the effects of recent rainfall, you may find the trail partially under water. Duck under a large dead oak tree covered in resurrection fern as the trail winds its way through the floodplain. The loblolly pines throughout this forest are of significant size. You walk over a small plank bridge crossing a drainage ditch.

Big steps lead up into an abandoned tree stand as the trail gains a little elevation and works its way between the oaks. By 2.1 miles the trail reaches a pair of log benches and drops into the cypress floodplain. The watermarks on the cypress trunks tell the story: this area can be 2 feet or more deep in water at times. If you encounter standing water here, you may wish to turn back. We saw stacks of lumber indicating plans for a boardwalk or bog bridge through the cypress strand in the future. Meanwhile, a few planks are laid down to get you through and around the muckier spots among the cypress knees. Dry spots may be thick with poison ivy.

Transitioning into a grassy area beyond the cypress strand, the trail rises up onto higher ground with water oaks and laurel oaks. At 2.5 miles you step into a clearing at the end of the trail, a small bluff above Prairie Creek. A picnic table provides a place to sit and enjoy the tannic creek, which flows slowly beneath a canopy of cypresses, rounding a bend. After visiting this serene spot, retrace your journey along the orange blazes back through the cypress strand and floodplain forest. You return to the junction with the Susan Wright Trail after 3.5 miles. Turn right. The trail leads you into uplands, a mix of pines and cabbage palms. A clearing on the left has a picnic table under the tall oaks. Deer trails lead into the woods. Stick to the obvious path, following the white blazes. The woods draw close to provide shade, with skinny cabbage palms towering overhead. Massive, whorled trunks of live oaks are swaddled in resurrection fern, resplendent after a rain. Bluestem palm grows throughout the understory.

The habitat transitions into an upland hammock with highbush blueberry, sparkleberry, and horse sugar beneath oak and sweetgum. The trail twists and winds through it, leading up to the pine plantation. A series of bog bridges cross a low swale where water can drain at times; however, they sometimes float to the side. Winding its way through pine plantations, the trail reaches the junction with the Yellow Trail at 4.1 miles, completing the loop. Continue straight ahead, following the white blazes, to retrace your route back to the parking area, completing the 4.7-mile hike.

Nearby Attractions

Stop at Pearl Country Store for locally grown produce, Florida books, and mouth-watering barbecue: **pearlcountrystore.com.** Rent canoes and kayaks for exploring Prairie Creek and Newnans Lake at Kate's Fish Camp, a decades-old outdoor destination: **katesfishcamp.com.** The Gainesville–Hawthorne State Trail provides a 16-mile ride each way between termini: **floridastateparks.org/gainesville-hawthorne.**

Directions

From I-75, Exit 374, Micanopy, drive east on CR 234 toward US 441. Turn south on US 441 and take it to the blinker in Micanopy at Pearl Country Store. Turn left on CR 234. Follow it north 6.8 miles to where it crosses the Gainesville–Hawthorne State Trail. Turn left and park in the parking area adjoining the rail-trail.

13

San Felasco Hammock Preserve State Park:

Moonshine Creek Trails

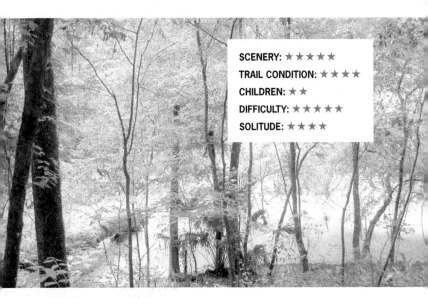

SCENERY: ★ ★ ★ ★ ★

TRAIL CONDITION: ★ ★ ★ ★

CHILDREN: ★ ★

DIFFICULTY: ★ ★ ★ ★ ★

SOLITUDE: ★ ★ ★ ★

LOOKING DOWN INTO CREEK SINK

GPS TRAILHEAD COORDINATES: N29° 42.858' W82° 27.653'

DISTANCE & CONFIGURATION: 2.5-mile balloon

HIKING TIME: 1.5 hours

HIGHLIGHTS: Appalachian-style ravines and wildflowers, enormous trees, sinkholes

ACCESS: Daily, 8 a.m.–sunset. Entrance fee: $2 per pedestrian or cyclist; $4 per vehicle.

MAPS: USGS *Gainesville West,* at trailhead kiosk

FACILITIES: Portable toilet and shaded picnic benches at trailhead, benches along the trails

WHEELCHAIR ACCESS: None

COMMENTS: Leashed dogs welcome. Bicycles are not permitted. Portions of the trail may flood at times. Trailhead shared with Hike 14, North Hiking Trails.

CONTACTS: San Felasco Hammock Preserve State Park: 386-462-7905; **floridastate parks.org/sanfelascohammock.** Friends of San Felasco Hammock: **sanfelasco.net.**

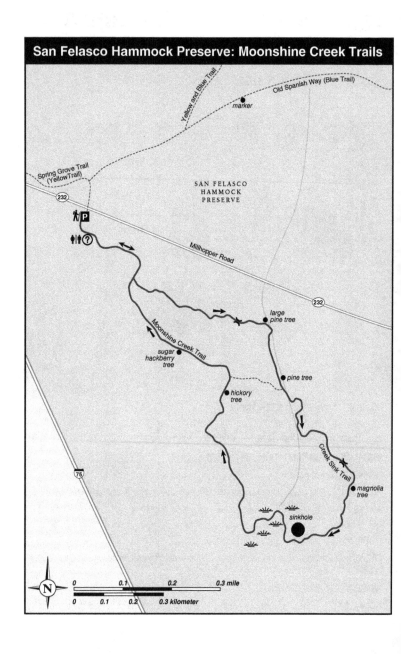

San Felasco Hammock Preserve: Moonshine Creek Trails

Yellow and Blue Trail

Old Spanish Way (Blue Trail)

● marker

Spring Grove Trail
(YellowTrail)

232

SAN FELASCO
HAMMOCK
PRESERVE

Millhopper Road

232

● large
pine tree

Moonshine Creek Trail

sugar ●
hackberry
tree

● pine tree

● hickory
tree

Creek Sink Trail

75

● magnolia
tree

sinkhole

N

| 0 | 0.1 | 0.2 | 0.3 mile |

| 0 | 0.1 | 0.2 | 0.3 kilometer |

Overview

At San Felasco Hammock, the trails on the south side of Millhopper Road immerse you in the botanical beauty and karst weirdness that are important facets of this state park protecting more than 7,300 acres northwest of downtown. Throughout Gainesville, creeks vanish into the ground, becoming part of the Floridan Aquifer. Along the two short but rugged trails that comprise this loop—Moonshine Creek Trail and Creek Sink Trail—you'll see the lush vegetation that grows along Moonshine Creek, as well as enormous deciduous trees in a forest surrounding the marshy sinkhole that swallows the creek.

Route Details

From the parking area, pass the picnic pavilion and privy, following the trail to a kiosk with park information and maps. Continue down the trail to a T intersection and turn right. Follow the broad, needle-strewn path into the slightly rolling hills topped with turkey oaks and pines, classic sandhill habitat. Passing a cluster of very short chinquapin oaks with serrated leaves, the trail sweeps to the right, entering a forest dense with laurel oaks. At a quarter mile, a sign guides you to the left, starting the loop.

Following the Moonshine Creek Trail, you quickly descend into the deciduous forest on a narrow, steep, and rooty footpath into the ravine. Sugarberry, hackberry, and oak tower overhead in a layered canopy. The understory is thick and vine-tangled, noisy with birds. Poison ivy and Virginia creeper send tendrils across the forest floor. It's an almost continuous descent; roots form a staircase in one spot. Past an arrow marker, the landscape falls off precipitously into one of the sinkholes. A beaten path leads down to its edge for a look. Continue along the main trail, which levels out and becomes sandy underfoot as you enter the floodplain of Moonshine Creek. You see an arrow marker in a yellow circle, the blaze for this loop. The trail curves past a large swamp chestnut oak, passing another sink with a fallen tree partially obscuring it.

At 0.6 mile you reach a bridge over Moonshine Creek, where wildflowers more commonly associated with the Appalachians thrive, including trillium and jack-in-the-pulpit. Clear and sand-bottomed, the stream sluices its way through the forest. After you cross the bridge, it's a climb uphill past some limestone-loving spleen-wort ferns. Crossing a swale where an ephemeral stream flows, you see a pond inside a sinkhole with mucky shores where raccoons have left their tracks. The trail curves away from the pond, climbing uphill. To the left, you can see that the landscape drops off in the distance. Sundial lupine carpets the forest floor.

Passing a cluster of needle palms dappled in sunlight, the trail curves and comes up to the base of a massive slash pine with an odd indent to its trunk, as if an elephant had leaned on it. Look up. You can hardly find the crown of the tree against the sky, it's that tall. Dropping off this small ridge, the trail descends into the floodplain

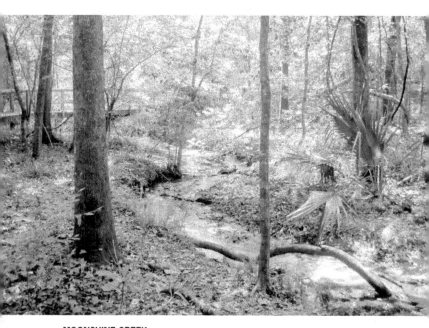

MOONSHINE CREEK

again to meet its junction with Creek Sink Trail at 0.8 mile. You see a bridge over Moonshine Creek on the right. Turn left.

Creek Sink Trail is the lesser traveled of the two loops, marked with faded orange blazes and newer red discs with arrows on them. Very little sunlight gets through the canopy, so mosquitoes are prevalent. The trail drops down into a rooty and sometimes wet part of the floodplain before scrambling to the top of a small limestone ridge, where trillium grows along the slope. Dropping steeply back down into the floodplain, you walk amid cinnamon fern and bluestem palm, passing a thick steel cable, a remnant from the past that mimics the coils of a nearby grapevine. Passing through a stand of young spruce pines, the trail descends past many trees of significant size. You cross a bridge over an ephemeral stream at 1.1 miles, with a willow marsh to the right. The trail ascends sharply, climbing a steep bluff through a slope forest past an enormous Southern magnolia. Looking down toward the marsh, you realize that you're inside a giant sinkhole and the marsh is in its bottom. This is Creek Sink, the end of the line for Moonshine Creek. A short side trail leads to an overlook above the sink.

Leaving the viewpoint, the trail climbs steeply uphill to a spot where, when it rains, water pours down the slope, creating a messy, muddy spot where water cascades into the sinkhole. As the trail turns, it shows off how precipitously the forest drops toward the bottom of the sink before leading you on a rapid descent. It feels like a hike in the Southern Appalachians, and increasingly so as the habitat shifts from slope forest to a deciduous forest with trees of increasingly amazing proportions. Flattening out a little, the trail provides another perspective of the willow marsh in the sinkhole.

Walking beneath tall sweetgum and hickory, you curve around the edge of the bottom of the big sink at its shoreline. Following the edge of the willow marsh briefly, you can see open water in the middle of the sink. Turning away from the sink, the trail begins its climb upward into the deciduous forest. The distant hum you hear is I-75. As you cross a small floodplain, make your way carefully across by stepping along spreading roots of large red maple trees. Climbing up a slope, the path heads directly between the bases of two very tall pines. The immense trunk on the right belongs to a tree more than 100 feet tall; we think it's an eastern hop hornbeam. The trail zigzags past numerous large deciduous trees on this steep slope, including sugar hackberry and pignut hickory, before it flattens out again. Just beyond the next trail marker is a brown sign. You've reached a T intersection with the Moonshine Creek Trail after 2 miles. Turn left.

After a slight uphill, you see a yellow blaze confirming you're back on the main trail. The trail flattens out and you start to hear traffic on Millhopper Road. The dense forest breaks up a little; you see laurel oaks and slash pines as the path broadens. At a trail junction, an old forest road comes in from the left, and a sign points to the exit. Passing the trail on the right, the descent you took earlier into the ravine at Moonshine Creek, you've completed the loop. Follow the broad path back to the trailhead to complete this 2.5-mile hike.

Nearby Attractions

The North Hiking Trails (Hike 14) leave from this same trailhead. Devil's Millhopper Geological State Park (Hike 4) is 4.2 miles east on Millhopper Road, and San Felasco Park (Hike 15) is nearby as well. To the north, Alachua has a quaint downtown with numerous eateries: **visitalachua.org.** Kids and adults alike will enjoy the Santa Fe Teaching Zoo at Santa Fe College: **sfcollege.edu/zoo.**

Directions

From I-75, Exit 390, take FL 222 (NW 39th Avenue) west 2.9 miles to CR 241 (NW 143rd Street). Turn right. Drive 2 miles north to Millhopper Road (NW 69th Avenue) and turn right. Continue 2 miles to the parking area on the south side of the road.

14

San Felasco Hammock Preserve State Park:
North Hiking Trails

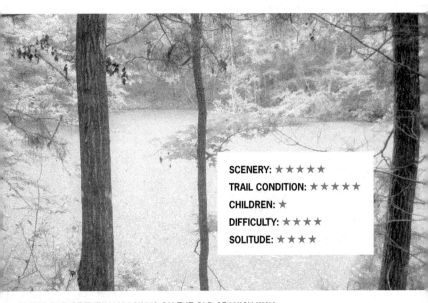

SCENERY: ★ ★ ★ ★ ★
TRAIL CONDITION: ★ ★ ★ ★ ★
CHILDREN: ★
DIFFICULTY: ★ ★ ★ ★
SOLITUDE: ★ ★ ★ ★

ALONG ONE OF THE MANY SINKS ON THE OLD SPANISH WAY

GPS TRAILHEAD COORDINATES: N29° 42.858' W82° 27.653'

DISTANCE & CONFIGURATION: 7.7-mile loop

HIKING TIME: 3.5 hours

HIGHLIGHTS: Rugged hills, karst landscapes, fabulous wildflowers

ACCESS: Daily, 8 a.m.–sunset. Entrance fee: $2 per pedestrian or cyclist; $4 per vehicle.

MAPS: USGS *Gainesville West*, at trailhead kiosk

FACILITIES: Portable toilet and shaded picnic benches at trailhead, benches along the trails

WHEELCHAIR ACCESS: None

COMMENTS: Leashed dogs welcome. Bicycles not permitted. Portions of the trail may flood at times. Trailhead shared with Hike 13, Moonshine Creek Trails.

CONTACTS: San Felasco Hammock Preserve State Park: 386-462-7905; **floridastate parks.org/sanfelascohammock.** Friends of San Felasco Hammock: **sanfelasco.net.**

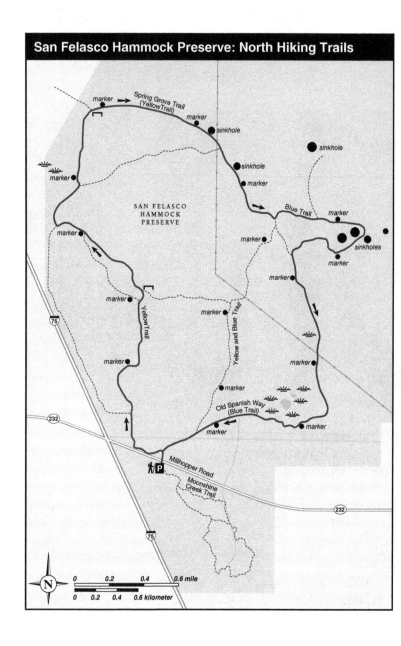

San Felasco Hammock Preserve: North Hiking Trails

Overview

Two major hiking trails comprise the North Hiking Trails (that is, north of Millhopper Road) at San Felasco Hammock Preserve State Park. The Spring Grove Trail creates a loop to the west, spending much of its time on hilly terrain in extensive sandhills. The Old Spanish Way—honoring the mission of San Francisco de Potano, which Spanish Jesuit priests established in this leafy forest in 1606—circles around karst features on the eastern side of the preserve. This hike follows the perimeter of the two trails clockwise and can be modified using the cross trails and forest roads to shorten this immersive 7.7-mile loop. Numbered markers throughout the loop help you determine where you are on the map.

Route Details

From the main parking area, carefully cross Millhopper Road—although there is a crosswalk and it is Florida law to stop for pedestrians, few drivers do. Walk up to a kiosk that marks the start of the loop. Although a sign directs you to the right, start your hike by turning left. Walking clockwise around the loop lets you deal with the hilliest terrain at the beginning of the hike and gets you past the short zone of traffic noise quickly so you can enjoy the solitude of the remainder of the hike.

Heading west on the yellow-blazed Spring Grove Trail, you parallel Millhopper Road. The trail passes a gate to the road as it curves right and starts downhill, trading traffic noise for the hum of I-75 as you drop past marker 11. After a big descent through the hardwood forest, a trail junction leads to an unmarked path to the left. Continue straight as the trail leads you uphill. Most of the trail system is the width of a forest road. To the right, the landscape drops off into the denser hammock below. As traffic noise fades away, you can clearly hear the sounds of birds. You see your first blaze with striping on it, which the park brochure says indicates the mileage along each of the two loops. Reroutes have changed the length of the trail, so these stripes aren't reliable.

These sandhills are relatively open, with alternating stretches of shade and sun. Loblolly and slash pine dominate, with tall hickories and the occasional Southern magnolia adding to the middle canopy, and younger oaks below. Beyond marker 10, you see a swale in the landscape that's likely a karst depression created by the collapse of limestone below the forest floor. You climb up and down the hills. Passing a ROAD CLOSED sign with marker 9 in front of it, turn right. Sweetgum, hickory, and dogwood grow among the oaks and pines.

At 1.4 miles you reach a bench at the junction with the Hammock Cutoff, one of several side trails that enable you to greatly trim the length of this loop. Turn left at this T intersection to stay on the perimeter trail. Wild white indigo blooms profusely in patches of grass beneath tall loblolly pines along this next stretch of trail. All of the trees in this part of the forest are huge, the hardwoods reminiscent of what you see along the Appalachian Trail in North Carolina. Part of the reason this state park exists is to protect the southernmost significant-sized stand of eastern deciduous forest in North America.

Just beyond a ROAD CLOSED sign, you walk past marker 8, heading uphill through the pine forest. In spring, the bright red spikes of coral bean in bloom stand out strongly against the new growth of the young oaks around it. Around 2.1 miles you start to hear traffic on the interstate again as the loop draws close to a corner of the property at a T intersection. Turn right, heading east and away from traffic noise. At an unmarked trail, you hear a sinkhole pond before you can see it hidden in the woods, as the frogs put on quite a chorus. Turn right to continue along the yellow blazes.

At 2.4 miles you reach the Sandhill Cutoff, a red-blazed trail headed east that cuts off a corner from the perimeter loop. Stay left to continue along the perimeter. Passing marker 7, the trail descends along the ecotone between sandhills and deciduous forest. At the next T intersection, there is a log bench. Turn right to stay on this loop. San Felasco Hammock Preserve spans more than 7,300 acres, with separate trail systems for equestrians and mountain bikers to the north. Forest roads that you encounter connect to other portions of the preserve.

Past marker 6 is a fork where a narrow path goes left. Stay with the main trail on the broader, road-width path. Ascending the next hill, you see young longleaf pines. Soon after a pretty cluster of dewberry, the trail reaches marker 5. In spring, large ivory-white blooms drape from the wooly pawpaw bushes. A dry sinkhole is on the right, with large trees and yucca rising from its bottom. Just beyond it, the trail passes under a power line at 3.7 miles, where the Sandhill Cutoff trail merges in. The trail heads downhill fast into the deep shade of the deciduous forest. An eerie hum fills the air as you draw close to a large sinkhole pond rich with amphibian life. A short side trail leads down to its rim. Ascending gently through the forest, you reach the Cross Trail junction at 4.2 miles. It's here that the Spring Grove Trail heads south. Stay on the outer perimeter by continuing straight ahead on the Old Spanish Way, marked with blue blazes.

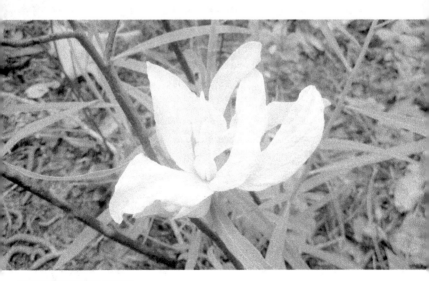

WOOLY PAWPAW IN BLOOM

The landscape drops off to a large sinkhole, evidenced by the lack of tree canopy above it. You reach a fork in the trail where the broad path you've been following curves to the left, and the blue blazes now lead you straight ahead into a hickory-dominated forest, past marker 12. Beneath a tightly knit canopy, the trail passes a sinkhole on the right framed by saw palmetto. From the watermark on a cypress, you can tell that the water levels fluctuate several feet, the sinkholes interconnected underground through the aquifer as there is no flowing surface water. With the many sinkholes along this next mile of trail, it's not safe to walk here if the trail is flooded.

The trail follows the rim of a bluff above the next water-filled sink, covered in a thick layer of green goo. Reaching a three-way junction of trails at 4.7 miles, turn right to round this sink. The trail narrows and becomes rooty underfoot. From a promontory over the sink, you can see a spruce pine rising from its far rim. Looking in every direction, you see more sinkholes and swales. The trail snakes its way through this fascinating karst landscape. Some of the sinks are shallow and small, and others are enormous, like the next one on the right, which looks like a giant pond. A path leads to its shore. Beyond it, the trail scrambles up a rocky slope, making a sharp left into a tunnel of vegetation. Passing marker 13, you see an old park sign in blue as the trail slowly rises to a higher elevation, back into the hickory-dominated forest. The narrow footpath ends at marker 14, reaching a T intersection with a forest road at 5.6 miles. Turn left.

Returning to sandhill habitat with a more open canopy, the trail is again a broad path with puddles of shade. Sand live oaks dominate, carpeting the footpath with crunchy leaves. You see deer moss and shiny lyonia as the path becomes sandy underfoot. Leaving this drier habitat, the trail reenters the hickory-dominated forest. Walking beneath the power line, you pass marker 15 as the forest gets darker and denser for a stretch, then enters an older patch of sandhills.

At a trail junction at 6.5 miles, turn right onto a footpath at a sign that says TRAILHEAD. The trail meanders between large saw palmetto and beneath tall sparkleberry within the deep shade of the hammock, and it just gets prettier as you reach marker 16. By 7 miles you emerge at a T intersection with a forest road. Turn right to continue through the hammock in dappled shade and sun. There are remnants of an old fence on the left.

The trail becomes a causeway above a patch of gum swamp before reaching marker 17, the last of the numbered markers around the loop. Climbing gently out of the deciduous forest, the trail enters its final stretch as a broad straightaway in the sun on a soft carpet of pine needles. At 7.4 miles you see a log bench at the junction with the Cross Trail, the second intersection of the two trails that make up the perimeter loop. Continue straight ahead on the Spring Grove Trail. The broad path narrows as you reach the trail kiosk, completing the loop. Turn left to exit. Crossing Millhopper Road, you complete the 7.7-mile hike.

Nearby Attractions

The rugged Moonshine Creek Trails (Hike 13) leave from this same trailhead. Devil's Millhopper Geological State Park (Hike 4) is 4.2 miles east on Millhopper Road, and San Felasco Park (Hike 15) is nearby as well. To the north, Alachua has a quaint downtown with numerous eateries: **visitalachua.org.** Dudley Farm Historic State Park provides a walk back in time on an authentic old Florida homestead: **floridastateparks.org/dudleyfarm.**

Directions

From I-75, Exit 390, take FL 222 (NW 39th Avenue) west 2.9 miles to CR 241 (NW 143rd Street). Turn right. Drive 2 miles north to Millhopper Road (NW 69th Avenue) and turn right. Continue 2 miles to the parking area on the south side of the road.

San Felasco Park

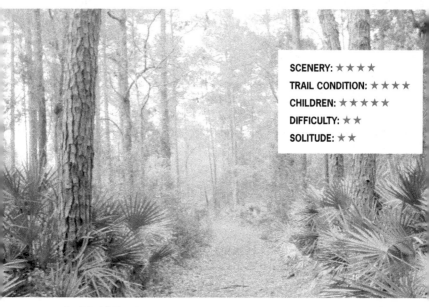

SCENERY: ★ ★ ★ ★
TRAIL CONDITION: ★ ★ ★ ★
CHILDREN: ★ ★ ★ ★ ★
DIFFICULTY: ★ ★
SOLITUDE: ★ ★

PINE FOREST SURROUNDING THE MAIN TRAIL

GPS TRAILHEAD COORDINATES: N29° 42.761' W82° 23.521'

DISTANCE & CONFIGURATION: 2-mile balloon

HIKING TIME: 45 minutes

HIGHLIGHTS: Cypress strand, cypress-lined Blues Creek

ACCESS: November–April: daily, 8 p.m.–6 p.m. May–October: daily, 8 a.m.–8 p.m. Free.

MAPS: USGS *Gainesville West,* on trailhead kiosk

FACILITIES: Restrooms, picnic area, and playground at the parking area; interpretive shelter at trailhead with overview of habitats in the park

WHEELCHAIR ACCESS: Use the paved bike path leading west from the parking area. Access is possible with minor assistance on the Main Trail, as the footpath is well groomed.

COMMENTS: Pets welcome. Strollers are most suitable on the Main Trail, the Marsh Trail, the Cypress Dome Trail, and the bicycle path. Bicycles are permitted on all trails. Not all of the trails shown on the map are marked at trail junctions.

CONTACTS: City of Gainesville Department of Parks, Recreation and Cultural Affairs, Nature Operations Division: 352-334-5067; **natureoperations.org**; **facebook.com/cityof gainesvillenature**

San Felasco Park

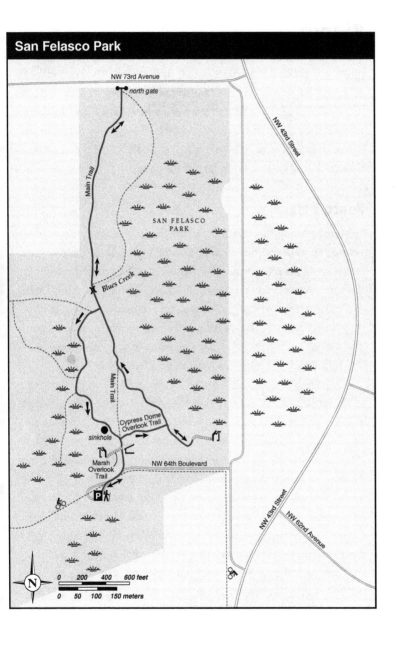

NW 73rd Avenue

north gate

NW 43rd Street

Main Trail

SAN FELASCO
PARK

Blues Creek

Main Trail

Cypress Dome
Overlook Trail

sinkhole

Marsh
Overlook
Trail

NW 64th Boulevard

P

NW 43rd Street

NW 62nd Avenue

N

| 0 | 200 | 400 | 600 feet |
| 0 | 50 | 100 | 150 meters |

Overview

On the north edge of Gainesville, San Felasco Park, opened in 2009, provides recreationists a place to play in the woods amid sometimes-wet pine flatwoods. With connections to nearby neighborhoods, it provides nicely shaded paths for walkers, runners, and residents walking their dogs. The biggest surprises along the park's trails are Blues Creek, a cypress-lined waterway, and a ribbon of cypress strand that marks the eastern boundary of the park.

Route Details

To start your hike, backtrack down the bike path toward the building you saw from the entrance road before you reached the parking area. A sign along the road at that point says MAIN TRAIL. The building is the Interpretive Shelter, containing information about the habitats you'll find in this park, and an overall park map. We're not sure if the map is an accurate representation of the trail system or reflects future plans, as we could not find signage for many of the trails shown on it. This hike covers the more obvious, easy-to-follow trails.

Leaving the back end of the shelter, follow the path back to the Main Trail, and cross it to take the Marsh Overlook Trail, a short boardwalk that leads out to a marshy pond surrounded by pine forest. Return to the Main Trail and turn left. Walk up to the CYPRESS DOME OVERLOOK TRAIL sign, and turn right. You meander through a high, dry forest of pines and oaks with clumps of saw palmetto, descending as you reach a boardwalk. Trail's end is an observation deck within a cypress strand. You can tell that the strand has been dry for a very long time, as large pine trees have intruded among the cypress. With residential development pressing up against this area, the hydrological flow across the landscape has been changed. Time will tell if these cypresses can survive without the water that once nourished them.

Turn around and backtrack along the boardwalk to the footpath again. Keep alert for the Cypress Trail, which is unmarked and leads you straight ahead where a jog in the Cypress Dome Overlook Trail goes to the left. The trail winds through the pine flatwoods within sight of the cypress strand. In winter, the cypresses stand out sharply against the rest of the forest because of their lack of needles.

After a half mile, you emerge at the Main Trail. Turn right. Walking through the upland forest of oaks and pines, you can still see the cypresses through the woods to your right. An unmarked trail junction goes off to the left; continue straight. The canopy thins. Slash pine and laurel oaks dominate the forest. Passing the next unmarked trail junction, continue straight.

The trail crosses a broad bridge over Blues Creek. It's a beautiful, narrow waterway hemmed in on both sides by tall cypress and rimmed with ferns. Continue straight ahead. The trail broadens and gains a little elevation as it enters a mature pine forest with a thick understory of saw palmetto. As the trail tunnels deeper into the pine forest, you start to see the backyards of homes in a subdivision to the left, a reminder that you are walking in an urban forest. The hum of traffic is minimal, drowned out by the birds.

After a mile the Main Trail ends at the park's north gate at NW 73rd Avenue. Turning around at this entrance, we noted a not-well-marked path to the left that might be the Flatwoods Trail North shown on the park map, but it was overgrown. Returning the way you came, you cross Blues Creek again at 1.4 miles. Immediately after the bridge, you have a decision to make: continue straight ahead on this broad path back to the trailhead (a 1.7-mile hike), or take the narrow path to the right to do a little exploring. Although shown on the map, the paths in this part of the park are not marked. Turning right, you immediately reach a trail junction; keep to the left. Walking among loblolly bay, slash pines, and highbush blueberry, you can tell the pine flatwoods can get soggy underfoot. To the right is a large marsh with an ephemeral pond in the middle. A trail comes in from the left; continue straight. Just beyond the marsh, you reach a Y intersection. Keep left, passing a depression to the left in a clearing between the pines.

At the T intersection that comes up next at 1.6 miles, wander off to the right a little ways, where there is a good view of a small depression marsh with standing water. Songbirds love this area. The trail ends abruptly in this direction at the boggy edge of the marsh. Backtrack to the T intersection, and continue straight across it to continue on the Pond Trail. Winding through the oaks and pines, it passes a water-filled depression, probably a sinkhole. A few moments later, the Pond Trail ends at the Main Trail, within view of the Cypress Dome Overlook Trail entrance. Turn right to exit and walk back to the parking area, wrapping up a 2-mile hike.

Nearby Attractions

Kids and adults alike will enjoy the Santa Fe Teaching Zoo at Santa Fe College: **sfcollege.edu/zoo.** With tours available by appointment only, the Lubee Bat Conservancy, a working conservation center, is a fascinating place to learn about fruit bats: **batconservancy.org.** San Felasco Park sits just north of Devil's Millhopper Geological State Park (Hike 4).

Directions

From I-75, Exit 390, take FL 222 east 3.4 miles to NW 43rd Street. Turn left. Continue 1.5 miles, crossing over Millhopper Road before you make a left at the brown sign for SAN FELASCO PARK at the curve in the road. Follow this road north past Cox Cable and a television station to enter the park. The road makes a sharp left into the park and continues back to end at a loop in the woods with parking spots, a playground, a picnic area, bike path access, and restrooms. The street address is 6400 NW 43rd Way.

Sweetwater Preserve

SCENERY: ★ ★ ★ ★
TRAIL CONDITION: ★ ★ ★ ★ ★
CHILDREN: ★ ★ ★ ★
DIFFICULTY: ★ ★ ★
SOLITUDE: ★ ★

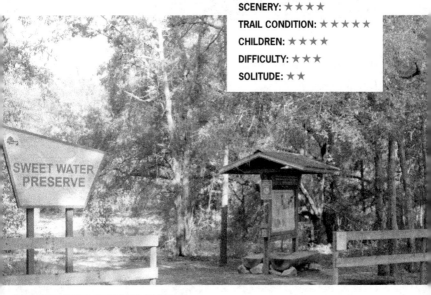

ENTRANCE TO SWEETWATER PRESERVE

GPS TRAILHEAD COORDINATES: N29° 37.267' W82° 18.450'

DISTANCE & CONFIGURATION: 2-mile balloon

HIKING TIME: 45 minutes

HIGHLIGHTS: Ravines, creek, wildflowers in spring and fall

ACCESS: November–April: daily, 7 a.m.–7 p.m. May–October: daily, 7 a.m.–8 p.m. Free.

MAPS: USGS *Micanopy*, on kiosk at preserve entrance

FACILITIES: Restrooms inside historic Bouleware Springs Waterworks, benches and interpretive information along the trail

WHEELCHAIR ACCESS: Only along the Gainesville–Hawthorne Trail connector to the preserve

COMMENTS: Pets welcome. Though the preserve is supposed to be hiking only, you may encounter cyclists cutting through from the mountain bike trails on the western side of the preserve.

CONTACTS: City of Gainesville Department of Parks, Recreation and Cultural Affairs, Nature Operations Division: 352-334-5067; **natureoperations.org**; **facebook.com/cityof gainesvillenature** (for trailhead area). Gainesville–Hawthorne State Trail: 352-466-3397; **floridastateparks.org/gainesville-hawthorne.** Alachua County Environmental Protection Department, Land Conservation Division: 352-264-6800; **alachuacounty.us.**

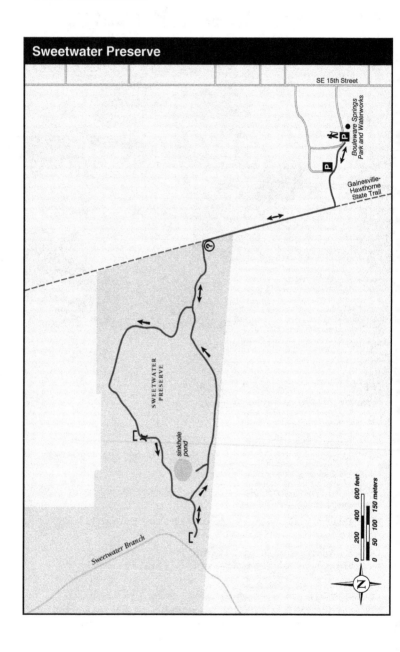

Sweetwater Preserve

SE 15th Street

Boulware Springs
Park and Waterworks

P

P

Gainesville-
Hawthorne
State Trail

SWEETWATER
PRESERVE

sinkhole
pond

Sweetwater Branch

600 feet
400
200
0

150 meters
100
50
0

N

Overview

Encompassing 125 acres bounded by Paynes Prairie and the Gainesville–Hawthorne State Trail, Sweetwater Preserve provides a buffer for the lower reaches of Sweetwater Branch, a stream that starts north of downtown and spends much of its time buried in culverts, draining stormwater from roadways. Inside the preserve, the waterway sparkles through the deep shade of a bluff forest, one of eight natural communities found along the hiking trail. The trick: finding Sweetwater Preserve, as its entrance is not at a trailhead but accessed via a popular bike trail.

Route Details

The hike begins at Bouleware Springs Park and Historic Waterworks near the waterworks around the spring basin. Walk uphill and through a gap in the fence at a sign that says GAINESVILLE–HAWTHORNE TRAIL, and continue uphill, looking for the next gap in the fence toward a parking area. Primarily for equestrian use, this is an alternate place to park but is farther from the restrooms and picnic area. Walk up to the large kiosk and the intersection with the paved Gainesville–Hawthorne State Trail. Turn right.

Since this is a cyclist-friendly city, the bike trail tends to be busy. Walk on the right side of the path and keep alert for passing cyclists. Just past the fence marking the boundary of Paynes Prairie Preserve State Park, you'll see the entrance to Sweetwater Preserve at 0.4 mile. Turn left to walk up to the kiosk; grab a map and sign in. Notice the bike rack? It's here to encourage cyclists to leave their bikes here and take a hike, but it's also a teaching tool. Painted to compare a coral snake—Florida's most venomous viper—with its mimic, a king snake, it makes for a great photo op.

Start down the footpath, which is defined by logs along its edge as it enters a patch of scrub amid scattered sand live oaks. You'll see showy clusters of lady lupine blooming here in spring. The Y intersection in the trail is the beginning of the loop. Although the trail marker directs you to the left, turn right to walk counterclockwise around the loop. This lets you experience the sunnier uplands first. The sand is soft underfoot. Deer moss thrives on this bright sand in puddles of shade under the oaks.

Before this land was a preserve, it was used for cattle grazing and farming, obvious from the old furrows. The trail winds along the edge of an open sandhill habitat under restoration to longleaf pine and wiregrass. Wooly pawpaw shows off its cream-colored blooms each spring. Strolling through a hardwood hammock along the edge of a mossy area, you're corralled onto the footpath by rotting logs of laurel oak resplendent with funky fungi. You can see the back side of the historic Pine Grove Cemetery, with healthy longleaf pines along the boundary.

At 0.8 mile the trail makes an abrupt left. Turning your back to the fence line, you plunge into a shady hardwood hammock. The trail heads down a gradual slope lined in cabbage palms. A bridge crosses over an ephemeral stream that drains a baygall—a small swamp of loblolly bay trees—in a sinuous path toward the creek. You can see through the trees on the left to the edge of a willow marsh in the bottom of a large sinkhole. Loblolly pines tower overhead.

The trail curves and comes to a T intersection at a sign that says CREEK. Turn right and follow this short, winding spur trail to where it ends at a bench above Sweetwater Creek. It's a clear, sand-bottomed stream, beautiful to behold. However, you don't want to go wading in it or drinking it. Its headwaters are downtown, so all of the water from city streets—plus treated sewage effluent—pours into this creek on its way to Paynes Prairie. And the alligators from the prairie, the ones you see from the La Chua Trail (Hike 10), sometimes crawl up the creek and wait for fish to rocket past in the clear water. Best to stay on the bluff.

Leaving the creek the way you came, you head uphill and pass the trail junction, walking through a dense stand of Southern magnolia. When you reach the next trail intersection, turn left at the sign that says THE POND. This short spur trail drops down the hill quickly to a bench overlooking a sinkhole pond thick with Virginia willow. There is a warning about alligators. You probably won't see any here, but in Florida, any body of water might have an alligator in it.

Scramble back uphill and continue straight ahead on the main trail, which meets up with and parallels the state park fence on the right. Yaupon holly grows thickly beneath the oaks and sweetgum shading this path. Pulling away from the fence, the trail turns left into a corridor flanked by oaks, some of which sport fuzzy mantles of resurrection fern. Continuing its gentle uphill climb, the trail reaches the end of the loop after 1.5 miles.

Continue straight ahead to exit the preserve, passing the kiosk and bike rack on your way out. Turn right and follow the paved Gainesville–Hawthorne State Trail back to the BOULEWARE SPRINGS CITY PARK sign. Turn left. Past the kiosk, head toward the wooden fence and follow it back around to the parking area at historic Bouleware Springs, completing a 2-mile hike.

Nearby Attractions

Upstream, Sweetwater Branch flows beneath University Avenue in downtown Gainesville past the Matheson Museum, the region's premier history museum: **mathesonmuseum.org.** A restored Mediterranean Revival–style hotel, the Thomas Center is a cultural venue with art galleries and gardens: **gvlculturalaffairs.org.** This part of Gainesville is home to the Southeast Historic Bed & Breakfast District with a bevy of B&Bs to choose from, including the Sweetwater Branch Inn: **sweetwaterinn.com.**

Directions

From I-75, Exit 382, drive east on SE Williston Road (FL 331), crossing US 441 after 4.3 miles. Continue around the curve past the western entrance to the preserve and the traffic light. Turn right onto SE Fourth Street, which curves slightly to become SE 21st Avenue. Turn right on SE 15th Street and continue a half mile to the park entrance. The first, easy-to-miss entrance leads to the equestrian-friendly parking lot nearest the trail; the main entrance leads to the parking lot near the historic waterworks, spring, and restrooms.

17 Tuscawilla Preserve

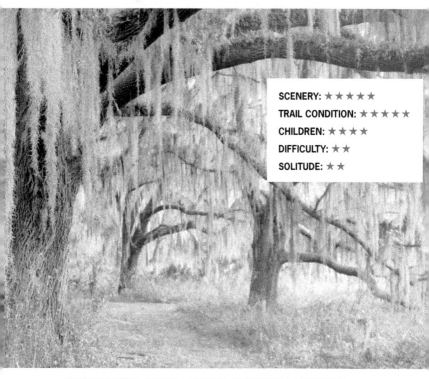

SCENERY: ★ ★ ★ ★ ★
TRAIL CONDITION: ★ ★ ★ ★ ★
CHILDREN: ★ ★ ★ ★
DIFFICULTY: ★ ★
SOLITUDE: ★ ★

UNDER THE MOSS-DRAPED LIVE OAKS OF TUSCAWILLA PRESERVE

GPS TRAILHEAD COORDINATES: N29° 30.151' W82° 16.178'

DISTANCE & CONFIGURATION: 0.7-mile loop

HIKING TIME: 20 minutes

HIGHLIGHTS: Ancient live oaks draped in Spanish moss, panoramas of Tuscawilla Prairie

ACCESS: Daily, sunrise–sunset. Free.

MAPS: USGS *Micanopy,* on trailhead kiosk

FACILITIES: Picnic tables under the oaks

WHEELCHAIR ACCESS: None

COMMENTS: Pets welcome, but bicycles not allowed. Future plans are for a boardwalk out into Tuscawilla Prairie. Be cautious of red ant nests and poison ivy if you step off the footpath into denser vegetation.

CONTACTS: Alachua Conservation Trust: 352-373-1078; **alachuaconservationtrust.org**

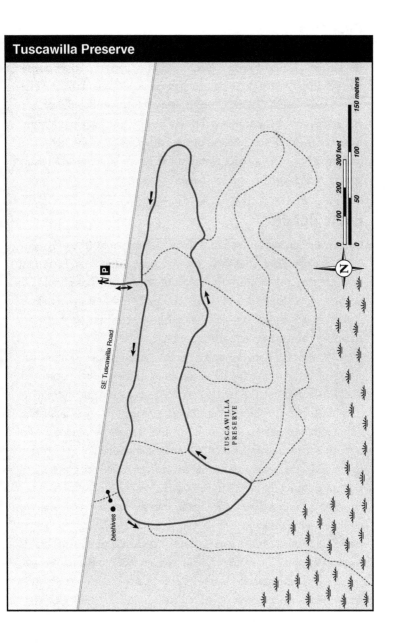

Tuscawilla Preserve

Overview

Acquired in 2006 by the Florida Communities Trust and managed by the Alachua Conservation Trust, Tuscawilla Preserve encompasses more than 500 acres along Tuscawilla Prairie. A former lake, the prairie is a large wetland along the southern edge of Florida's oldest interior settlement, Micanopy, established in 1821. Archaeologically and historically significant because of the native peoples who once lived along this basin, it's an excellent destination for birding and a beauty spot crowned with ancient live oaks.

Route Details

Cross over Tuscawilla Road to walk to the trail kiosk (the only place where the name Thrasher Park is used) and pick up a map. Turn right to begin the loop beneath the shade of ancient live oaks draped in Spanish moss. This is one of those trails that must be mowed to keep it clear, as it is very grassy and parklike under the oaks, enabling you to survey the scenery in every direction.

As the trail slips through a dense thicket of young palms, you see resurrection fern clinging to the limbs of the live oaks overhead. Stay to the right at the trail junction to remain on the outer loop. It parallels the not-so-busy road into Micanopy. You pass a bluebird box, a reminder to keep alert for birds. This is an excellent location for birding, with hundreds of sandhill cranes sometimes congregating in the open spaces, songbirds flitting between trees and tall grasses, and raptors scouting the wetlands for a meal.

At 0.2 mile a pass-through stile at a gate enables pedestrians to walk out to the road. The trail curves, soon surrounded by a thicket of blackberry bushes. As a mowed path, the trail heads out into the prairie itself, away from the treeline. An old wooden fence to the right marks the edge of where cows roamed before the prairie became conservation land. The prairie itself is a sea of tall grasses and dog fennel. Clusters of Florida myrtle peep out above the grasses. A path leaves the loop to the right (and might be the future boardwalk location), but the main trail, the broader path, curves back toward the live oak hammock. At a T junction in front of live oaks covered in Spanish moss, turn right.

The trail leaves the canopy of oaks just long enough to show off the gradation of grass heights along the prairie rim. You walk back into the shade along a grand corridor, enjoying the splendor of sunlight streaming through dense draperies of Spanish moss beneath oaks of incredible size. To the left, you can see the kiosk at the beginning of the loop. Reaching a T intersection with a cross trail to the kiosk at a half mile, you'll find a picnic bench. Turn right. The trail gets a little confusing, as two paths parallel the prairie's edge. Stick with the one closer to the treeline. The trail loops around through hardwood hammock, coming close to the property boundary again before bringing you back beneath the oaks toward the kiosk and picnic spot. Turn right at the kiosk to cross the road and return to the parking area.

Nearby Attractions

Take the time to see the burial mounds at Micanopy Native American Heritage Park, which shares this trailhead. With its antiques shops and art galleries, historic Micanopy is fun to visit, and you can't beat Aunt Sherry's Chicken Salad at Coffee and Cream: **micanopy coffeeshop.com.** Stop at the Micanopy Historical Society Museum for background on the peoples who lived along Tuscawilla Prairie: **afn.org/~micanopy.** Barr Hammock Preserve (Hike 2) and Paynes Prairie Preserve State Park: Wacahoota Trail (Hike 11) are just up the road.

Directions

From I-75, Exit 374, Micanopy, follow CR 234 east for 0.6 mile to NW Seminary Avenue. Turn right and drive 0.7 mile through the historic residential district to NE Cholokka Boulevard, which is flanked by the historic downtown. Turn right and continue along the road as it leaves town; drive another half mile to the parking area on the left at the Micanopy Native American Heritage Park.

University of Florida NATL Nature Trails

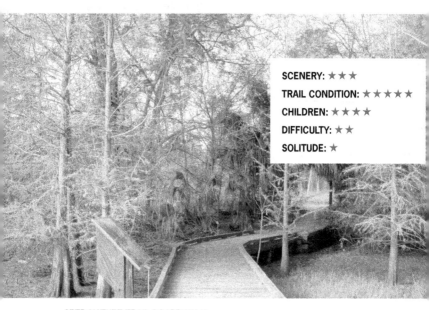

SCENERY: ★ ★ ★
TRAIL CONDITION: ★ ★ ★ ★ ★
CHILDREN: ★ ★ ★ ★
DIFFICULTY: ★ ★
SOLITUDE: ★

SEEP NATURE TRAIL BOARDWALK

GPS TRAILHEAD COORDINATES: N29° 38.091' W82° 22.191'

DISTANCE & CONFIGURATION: 1.5-mile loop

HIKING TIME: 45 minutes

HIGHLIGHTS: Extensive interpretive information, wetlands boardwalk

ACCESS: Daily, sunrise–sunset. Coin-metered parking; free parking in Entomology lot Monday–Friday after 3:30 p.m. and all day Saturday–Sunday and holidays (or 24/7 with UF decal).

MAPS: USGS *Gainesville East,* on trailhead kiosk. Detailed interpretive guides are available online: **natl.ifas.ufl.edu/naturetrails/history.php.**

FACILITIES: Kiosk at trailhead, benches and interpretive stations along the trail, picnic tables in the Natural Area Park along the SEEP Trail

WHEELCHAIR ACCESS: None

COMMENTS: Leashed pets welcome. No smoking. Bicycles not permitted on trails. Please stay on marked trails and do not disturb flagging/signage.

CONTACTS: natl.ifas.ufl.edu

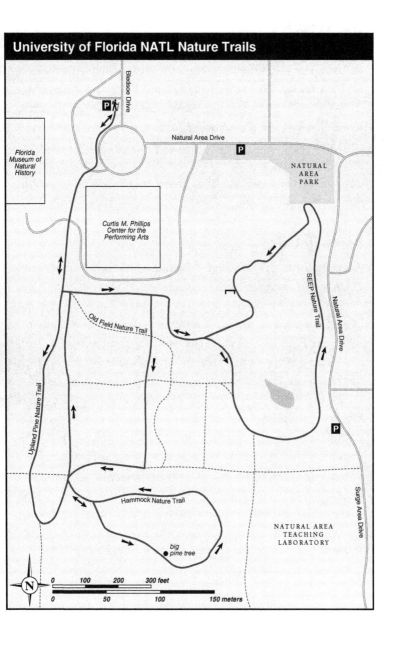

University of Florida NATL Nature Trails

Bledsoe Drive

P

Florida Museum of Natural History

Natural Area Drive

P

NATURAL AREA PARK

Curtis M. Phillips Center for the Performing Arts

SEEP Nature Trail

Natural Area Drive

Old Field Nature Trail

Upland Pine Nature Trail

P

Hammock Nature Trail

NATURAL AREA TEACHING LABORATORY

Surge Area Drive

big pine tree

N

| 0 | 100 | 200 | 300 feet |
| 0 | 50 | 100 | 150 meters |

Overview

Tucked behind the Florida Museum of Natural History and the Curtis M. Phillips Center for the Performing Arts, the University of Florida Natural Area Teaching Laboratory is an outdoor classroom where students and visitors can immerse themselves in several common Florida habitats and get to know them well, thanks to identification and interpretation of the habitats and their inhabitants. Although this 49-acre natural area is entirely surrounded by the bustle of Gainesville, it's an excellent launch point for learning plant identification before you head out to the quieter hikes in the region.

Route Details

From the front of the Florida Museum of Natural History, walk around the building to the left. You'll see a blue sign directing you to the nature trails. Walk downhill and across the access road to the back of the museum to reach the welcome kiosk. You can pick up a map here. Trails take off in several directions from this point. Turn left to follow the fence, passing a grid of small trails that intersect the Old Field Trail. The understory beneath the pines is entirely open.

Continue along the perimeter, passing a side trail. Songbirds flit through the trees and warble, calling attention to the fact that nearby traffic noise is not drowning out the sounds of nature. A kiosk on the left at 0.2 mile explains the purpose of the SEEP Nature Trail, showcasing the University's Stormwater Ecological Enhancement Project, a man-made wetland with gradients of marsh and swamp engineered to clean stormwater from the surrounding parking areas. A boardwalk is straight ahead, but the signs direct you to the right to start the loop. It's helpful to learn common Florida plants from the interpretive markers along it, such as wild radish and Cuban jute. As the trail passes another junction, there is a pond to the left. At a wide intersection, the SEEP Nature Trail turns left, passing the back side of several greenhouses and a warning sign about alligator nesting. Don't wander down that side trail to the pond.

Interpretive signage talks about inhabitants of this ecosystem, including cricket frogs and tree frogs, on the way to a back entrance to the trail system. The basin below is described as a self-organizing system, with 120 species of native plants thriving after restoration of the pond. Following the fence, the trail passes another back entrance after a half mile at the tiny Natural Area Park, a shady spot with picnic tables. It drops downhill past an array of interpretive signs about insects into the treatment marsh portion of the wetland area. The boardwalk begins, winding through giant cutgrass and marsh fern. The sound of burbling water is constant as you pass a small weir. The boardwalk curves into a shrubby swamp with a fringe of wild iris and wax myrtle, passes a cattail marsh, and enters a planted cypress swamp. On a small island, a bench adjoins a basket oak. Water flows slowly through this man-made series of wetlands down a natural slope to the alligator nesting pond, which is at the base of a gently sloped sinkhole. As the boardwalk ends, so does the loop.

Retrace your steps along the fence back to the first left, entering the Old Field Nature Trail at a sign that says OLD FIELD PLOT B.

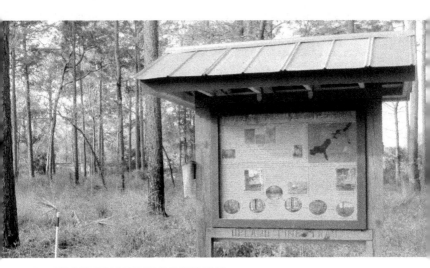

KIOSK AT THE START OF THE UPLAND PINE TRAIL

This grassy path leads uphill to the forested fringe beyond the field. With its roots as the Florida Agricultural College, this is part of the living laboratory for students at the University of Florida. Small signs sprout from the grasses under the pines, indicating how old that section of the field is—that is, how long it has been since it was last tilled, showing the natural succession of a field to a forest over time.

At a four-way junction, continue straight ahead beneath the slash pine through more succession plots. At the OLD FIELD NATURE TRAIL sign before a forest road along the edge of the woods, turn right. One interpretive marker you shouldn't ignore is poison ivy. It grows in many forms in Florida, from thick vines dangling overhead and mimicking hickory branches to this very common type, a vine in the grass.

As this trail ends, you reach the Hammock Trail kiosk at the edge of the denser forest at 0.8 mile. Turn left at the kiosk to start this loop, which enters an unrestored upland pine forest to show what happens as the forest goes through natural succession. At the fork, keep right. Notice how many laurel oaks there are? This is one of the more opportunistic trees in Florida and will take over an old field and turn it into a forest. According to the signs, this was a treeless field 65 years ago. Laurel oak forests tend to look scraggly, dense, and unkempt compared to the sandhill habitat that should be here.

The elevation drops as the trail enters an upland hammock. This is an excellent section of trail for learning about native Florida trees and plants, although the signage (like the words LOBLOLLY PINE strapped to whopping pine tree trunks) is intrusive at times. The footpath meanders and dips through a slightly undulating landscape with karst features, naturally sculpted by eroding limestone. The trail climbs up into the laurel oak forest to complete the loop, emerging at the Hammock Trail kiosk. You've hiked 1 mile.

At this junction of trails, walk straight ahead to the welcome kiosk at the entrance. Turn left to start the Upland Pine Trail, the final loop. It leads you through an "island of restoration" adjacent to homes on the edge of the University, amid what was once a farmer's field. Here, restoration to a healthy sandhill habitat, dominated by longleaf pine and wiregrass, is well underway. Thanks to the labels, you can compare the bark and needles of loblolly, slash, and longleaf pines to the leaves and bark of red oaks and turkey oaks. The farther you go on this trail, particularly once you cross the old forest road, the healthier the habitat looks. Leaving the pines, the trail loops left into the laurel oak forest and emerges next to the opposite side of the Hammock Trail kiosk.

Continue straight ahead down the path you've already trod between the pines and the old field. Reaching the welcome kiosk at the entrance gate, leave the preserve by walking straight ahead and up past the Florida Museum of Natural History to the parking lot, completing a 1.5-mile hike.

Nearby Attractions

Trail access is through the UF Cultural Complex, home to the Florida Museum of Natural History, a don't-miss museum for anyone interested in natural Florida. The museum includes a beautiful Butterfly Rainforest: **flmnh.ufl.edu.** Next door is the Samuel P. Harn Museum of Art: **harn.ufl.edu.** Just west of I-75 off Archer Road is Kanapaha Botanical Gardens, boasting 62 acres of gardens and Florida's largest collection of bamboo species: **kanapaha.org.**

Directions

From I-75, Exit 384, follow Archer Road east 1 mile to the intersection with SW 34th Street (FL 121). Turn left and continue 0.7 mile, past the Doyle Conner Center, to turn east onto Hull Road across from the Hilton. Turn right into the parking area just past the Harn Museum of Art. Park either in the flat-rate lot (currently $4) if you plan to do the hike and visit either or both of the museums, or use a metered space (45-minute limit) and watch your time if you're just doing the hike.

19 # Watermelon Pond Preserve

SCENERY: ★ ★ ★ ★ ★
TRAIL CONDITION: ★ ★ ★
CHILDREN: ★ ★ ★
DIFFICULTY: ★ ★ ★
SOLITUDE: ★ ★ ★ ★ ★

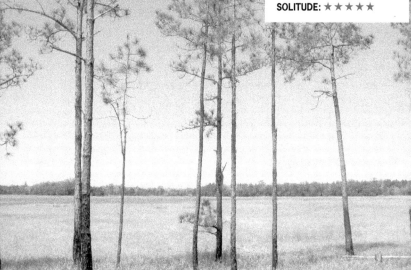

THE OPEN PRAIRIE OF WATERMELON POND

GPS TRAILHEAD COORDINATES: N29° 33.348' W82° 36.423'

DISTANCE & CONFIGURATION: 5.5-mile balloon

HIKING TIME: 2.5 hours

HIGHLIGHTS: Panoramic views of vast prairie ecosystems, wildlife sightings

ACCESS: Daily, sunrise–sunset. Free.

MAPS: USGS *Archer*, at trailhead kiosk

FACILITIES: Picnic tables at the trailhead under the oaks

WHEELCHAIR ACCESS: None

COMMENTS: Leashed pets welcome. Trails shared with equestrians and cyclists. Seasonal hunting is permitted. Check hunting dates in advance at **myfwc.com.**

CONTACTS: Florida Fish and Wildlife Conservation Commission, North Central Region: 386-758-0525; **myfwc.com.** Alachua County Environmental Protection Department: 352-264-6800; **alachuacounty.us** (trailhead).

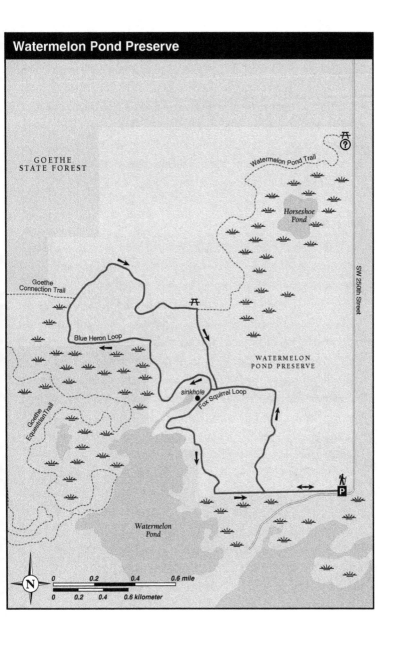

Watermelon Pond Preserve

GOETHE
STATE FOREST

Watermelon Pond Trail

Horseshoe
Pond

Goethe
Connection Trail

Blue Heron Loop

WATERMELON
POND PRESERVE

sinkhole

Fox Squirrel Loop

Goethe
Equestrian Trail

SW 250th Street

P

Watermelon
Pond

N

| 0 | 0.2 | 0.4 | 0.6 mile |
| 0 | 0.2 | 0.4 | 0.6 kilometer |

Overview

On the westernmost edge of Alachua County, Watermelon Pond is a sprawling prairie complex that was once an extensive lake, a haven for wading birds. Changes in population density and water usage dried up the landscape years ago, leaving only a fraction of the water behind. Protecting more than 4,200 acres, this is one of the more remote natural lands close to Gainesville. With panoramic views along miles of prairie rim, the 5.5-mile double-loop trail system is a delightful destination for hiking.

Route Details

Walk uphill to the kiosk, pick up a map, and head west down the trail. An arrow confirms your route. From this inauspicious and some-what boring start—a worn path between a firebreak and a fence—you wouldn't expect the beauty that lies beyond. After 0.4 mile the trail reaches the beginning of the Fox Squirrel Loop. Turn right and cross the firebreak to enter the sandhills. The trail is well named; we'd already seen three of these uncommon squirrels by the time we reached this point. The fox squirrel is much larger than a gray squirrel, with tawny chestnut fur, a dark mask around and above its eyes, and white fur around its nose. There are three subspecies in Florida, but the one you see here is the Sherman's fox squirrel, which has been designated a species of special concern.

The first blaze you see is on a strange quad-trunked loblolly pine. The trail is marked with a mixture of yellow blazes and sign-posts, but you have to watch for them. The next marker isn't obvious, but the path is. It skirts a low prairie on the right, dry and filled with blackberry bushes at its lowest point. Yellow jasmine drapes over the oaks on the hill. To the left are Florida rosemary bushes with deer moss and reindeer lichen at their bases, a smidgen of rosemary scrub.

After the trail curves left through a patch of forest, a yellow double blaze points you past another swale of prairie. Rosemary bushes grow at the edge of this prairie, along with deer moss and

134

sphagnum moss. A road vanishes into the woods on the far side. Stay to the left at the fork in the trail. Clusters of sandhill lupine grow in the low grasses, their pinkish-lilac blooms in evidence in late winter. Climbing through a patch of trees, you reach an open area. Fall wildflowers are particularly pretty through this section. Passing a pine with a catface, the trail curves to the left, just as it does each time you reach a point where you aren't quite sure where it goes.

You reach a T intersection at 1 mile. Turn left. The trail follows a firebreak—not the easiest of walking—as you climb up the next hill, passing an old pasture overgrown with dog fennel. Straight ahead is your first glimpse of the vast prairie of Watermelon Pond. The trail curves right, reaching a junction with the sign: NORTH PARKING /SOUTH PARKING. Turn left and walk down to the trail map. You're at the junction of the Fox Squirrel Loop and the Blue Heron Loop. Continue down the slope, through the rim of sand live oak along the prairie's edge, to the next marker. Turn right to start the Blue Heron Loop, also blazed yellow.

Walking along the expanse of prairie, you can see for quite some distance. After 1.7 miles you reach a trail intersection. Straight ahead is a short detour to a point with a view of what's left of Watermelon Pond. The Blue Heron Trail turns right. Follow it into the forest, where it works its way between rows of planted pines and large sand live oaks along another arm of the prairie. Leaving the shade, the trail pops out at a T intersection facing the prairie. Turn right. Passing a sign that says STATE FOREST BOUNDARY (you're on the edge of Goethe State Forest), the trail follows a forest road with soft sand in places. Reaching the next T intersection, at the corner of the prairie, turn left.

Following the yellow blazes down a sand road along the rim of the prairie, you pass a road into the woods on the right. The path broadens and becomes more of a firebreak for a stretch, leaving the prairie rim. After a short stretch of forest, you reach a Y junction with a trail going off to the prairie rim. Keep right. The trail sweeps sharply to the right to follow another arm of the prairie. By 2.7 miles the official connector trail to Goethe State Forest goes to the left at a sign, leading to a trailhead off County Road 337. It, too, is blazed yellow, which is confusing. Pass by it and continue straight ahead to stay on the Blue Heron Loop. The trail follows the prairie rim along patches of rosemary scrub. In the distance, a fence marks a boundary of the preserve. Curving to the right, the trail enters some woods before it emerges along another prairie, reaching a reverse Y intersection. Stay right, along the prairie rim, passing a path that goes off to the left as the trail starts to circle this prairie. At 3.4 miles a sand road goes into the woods on the right. Go straight, and you'll see the next confirmation blaze.

After meeting the path that crosses the prairie (a shortcut in the dry season), the trail curves right and uphill into a pretty sand live oak hammock. Crossing the next prairie, you see more forest on the other side. After 3.7 miles you reach a picnic area with covered picnic benches under the deep shade of live oaks. This spot marks the intersection with the Watermelon Pond Trail, which leads to the north (equestrian) trailhead. Make sure you make the right turn to continue on the Blue Heron Loop, south along an old road under a shady tree canopy. Popping out into the sunshine, the trail parallels a pine plantation for a short distance.

At the next junction with a sand road coming in from the right, there is a sign: NORTH PARKING/SOUTH PARKING. Make sure you're headed toward the South Parking area, walking along the edge of an old pasture. You reach the next sign at 4 miles. Turn right and walk down the slope, past the map, to the junction of the two trails again. You've completed the Blue Heron Loop.

Turn left at the trail junction to finish the second half of the Fox Squirrel Loop, which hugs the prairie rim. Two sand roads on the left lead uphill. As the road you're walking along sweeps uphill to the left, leave it to stay with the prairie rim. A marker points straight ahead. You're close enough to look into the prairie bottom, and it's quite interesting. Having been the bottom of a lake for so long, it is full of swales where water may still collect, with one deep sinkhole adjacent to the footpath.

Looking out over the prairie, it's an impressive view across a vast landscape, even more so than the panoramas of the Blue Heron Loop. Water sparkles in the distance in what is left of Watermelon Pond, way out in the middle of the grasslands at the heart of it all. As the trail curves left, the full extent of the expanse becomes visible. You see what looks like a dock and several homes in the distance. The trail curves with the prairie rim, reaching a fence. Here, after 4.6 miles, it turns left and heads uphill, staying within sight of the fence until it begins to follow it east. Climbing up and over a hill, which is part of a peninsula sticking out into the prairie, the trail continues down the slope, meeting the junction with the Fox Squirrel Trail at 5.1 miles. Continue straight ahead along the trail to exit, reaching the kiosk at the Watermelon Pond Park Trailhead after 5.5 miles.

Nearby Attractions

Newberry's quaint downtown is home to some fine eateries: **visit gainesville.com/nearby-towns/newberry.** The Archer Railroad Museum tells the Civil War tale of Yulee's railroad: **visitgainesville.com/attractions /archer-railroad-museum.** Experience living history at an original pioneer homestead farmed by several generations of the Dudley family: **floridastateparks.org/dudleyfarm.**

Directions

Take I-75, Exit 387, to follow FL 26 (Newberry Road) west 11.5 miles to Newberry. Turn south on US 27/41 and continue 2.9 miles to CR 28 (SW 46th Avenue). Turn right and drive west 1.2 miles to SW 250th Street. Turn left and drive south on SW 250th Street for 3.7 miles, passing the northern trailhead for Watermelon Pond en route. The road ends at Watermelon Pond Park. Park on the left when you enter the park; the right-hand side has deep, soft sand from horse trailers turning around in a low spot.

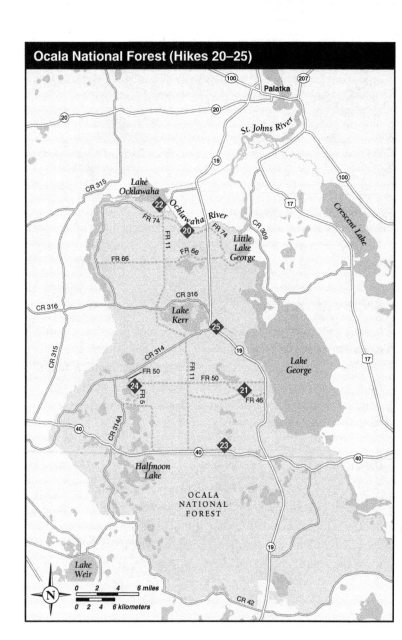

Ocala National Forest (Hikes 20–25)

Ocala National Forest

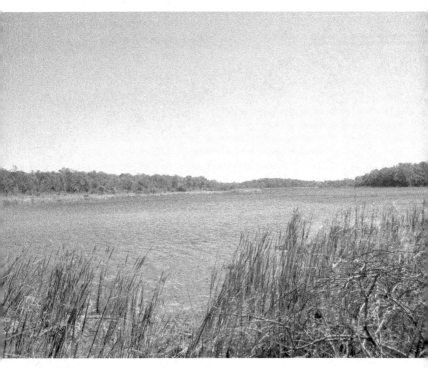

SALT SPRINGS RUN; *see Hike 25, page 172*

20 Davenport Landing Trail

SCENERY: ★ ★ ★ ★ ★
TRAIL CONDITION: ★ ★ ★
CHILDREN: ★ ★ ★
DIFFICULTY: ★ ★
SOLITUDE: ★ ★ ★ ★ ★

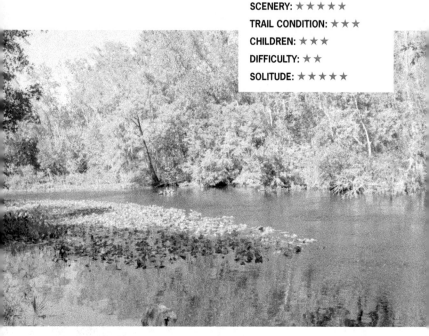

OCKLAWAHA RIVER AT DAVENPORT LANDING

GPS TRAILHEAD COORDINATES: N29° 28.336' W81 46.403'

DISTANCE & CONFIGURATION: 0.7-mile balloon

HIKING TIME: 30 minutes

HIGHLIGHTS: Views along the Ocklawaha River, archeological sites

ACCESS: Open 24/7. Free.

MAPS: USGS *Lake Delancy*, Ocala National Forest website

FACILITIES: Kiosks with interpretive information

WHEELCHAIR ACCESS: None

COMMENTS: Camping is not permitted at the landing. Consult the prescribed fire map on the forest website before entering the area. Paddlers can access the trail from the landing. Please do not disturb archaeological sites. Be aware of hunting seasons, and wear blaze orange if visiting during a hunt. FR 74 may be tough to drive after a rain.

CONTACTS: Ocala National Forest: 352-236-0288; **www.fs.usda.gov/ocala**

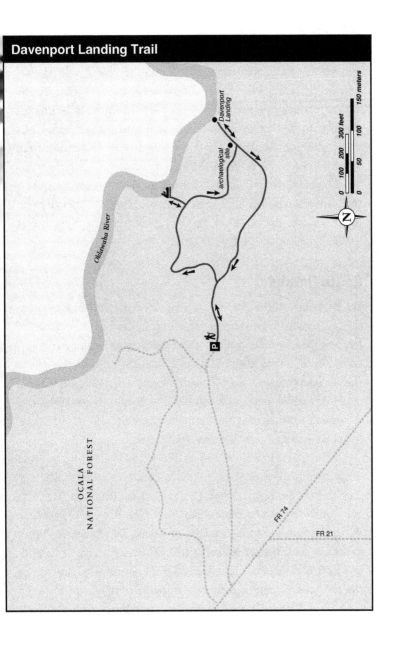

Davenport Landing Trail

Davenport
Landing

archaelogical
site

Ohlawaha River

OCALA
NATIONAL FOREST

FR 74

FR 21

0 100 200 300 feet

0 50 100 150 meters

P

Overview

The most obscure interpretive trail in the Ocala National Forest is well off the beaten path along the Ocklawaha River, accessed via a narrow dirt road. Why here? Location, location, location: in the 1800s, Florida's rivers served as highways to the interior. During the steamboat era, Davenport Landing was one of the last high bluffs that steamboats would pass as they made their way downriver from Silver Springs to the St. Johns River, 8 miles away. The landing master, Thomas Cassidy Fillyaw, is buried on the site, not far from a more ancient burial ground, the Davenport Mound. Although heavily looted over the centuries, in 1894 finds from the mound were declared to be up to 1,200 years old.

Route Details

The trail starts at the gate. Flanked by blueberries and bracken fern, this is a scrubby flatwoods habitat with shoulder-high saw palmetto, longleaf pine, and pond pine, which tends to grow along tributaries of the St. Johns River. A line of scrub oaks parallels the trail to the left, and you feel a slight downhill trend. After 400 feet, the trail reaches a marker that points to the left. Ill-defined at first because of infrequent maintenance, the footpath slips right into the scrub oak forest, down a tight corridor beneath the oaks.

The trail starts to drop sharply. Curving to the right to avoid dropping into the floodplain, it reaches an intermingling of habitats: bluff forest creeping into the Big Scrub, with tall Southern magnolia, pignut hickory, and American holly. To the left you can see water in the distance, beyond the cypresses of a floodplain forest. The break in the sky confirms you're almost at the Ocklawaha River. This sinuous river and its jungle-like floodplain shores attracted tourists by the boatload during the early days of Florida's statehood; the Hart Steamship Line built special, narrow steamboats to navigate its twisty, winding channels from its mouth at the St. Johns River to the hotel at Silver Springs.

Lined by switch cane, a native bamboo, a side trail leads down to the river. Take this trail for a walk right to the river's edge, keeping alert for alligators and snakes. By the watermarks on the surrounding cypress—up to 3 feet high—you can tell how much the river can rise after heavy rains near its source. One of several rivers in Florida that flow north, the Ocklawaha rises from a mosaic of wet pine flatwoods and cypress domes near Tampa called the Green Swamp, working its way toward the Ocala National Forest through a series of large lakes near Leesburg. Heavily disturbed by the Army Corps of Engineers around Moss Bluff (Hike 34, Ocklawaha Prairie Restoration Area) and Rodman Reservoir (Hike 22, Florida Trail: Rodman to Lake Delancy), its wild nature remains along a lengthy stretch outlining the western boundary of the Ocala National Forest.

Returning to the main trail, turn left. Large rusty lyonia—the tallest of the species are found in the Big Scrub—joins sand live oaks in shading the trail as you continue through the scrub forest. At 0.3 mile the trail reaches a junction with directional signs and two kiosks to the left. Step over to the leftmost kiosk, which adjoins Davenport Mound and explains its archaeological importance. Arrowheads found along these shores indicate humans settled here as early as 10,000 BC, living off the bounty of the forest and waterways.

The other kiosk explains steamboating on the Ocklawaha River, as you've reached the high bluff of Davenport Landing. A historic map shows the location of the many landings that steamboats would visit on their route to Silver Springs, as well as vividly named points for navigators to watch for, like Needle's Eye, Rough and Ready Cut, and Hell's Half Acre. As the last high bluff before northbound boats reached the St. Johns River, it was an important place to stock up on wood to feed the boilers.

From the kiosk, a series of steps lead down to the riverfront, where stonework and an old cypress log might have been used as part of the landing. It's a beauty spot, well worth your time for birding. The trail loops around and up the slope to the right. Once you climb back to the kiosk, take the other path under the live oaks at the PARKING sign.

Nicely framed by saw palmetto and gallberry, the trail corridor provides a good bit of shade as it follows the edge of the ecotone between scrubby flatwoods and oak scrub. The sugar white sand in the footpath shows imprints of many animals, especially raccoon and deer.

At a fork in the trail, keep left, walking between the pond pines. Within a few moments, you're back to the beginning of the loop. Continue straight ahead to exit, reaching the gate and parking area after a 0.7-mile walk.

Nearby Attractions

Ocklawaha Canoe Outpost can assist with rentals and shuttles for paddling this stretch of the Ocklawaha River and has campsites and cabins on the river: **outpostresort.com.** A unique piece of Florida history in motion, the Fort Gates Ferry crosses the St. Johns River north of Salt Springs: **bit.ly/fortgates.** Hike 22, Florida Trail: Rodman to Lake Delancy, can be accessed via FR 77 west to FR 11 north, although the road can get rough at times.

Directions

Driving 8.5 miles north from the intersection of CR 316 and FL 19 in Salt Springs, turn left off FL 19 onto FR 74 just before the Ocklawaha River bridge. FR 74 parallels the river in a northwesterly direction, and can be rough or soft sand in spots but accessible by most vehicles except after heavy rains. Drive 2.5 miles down the forest road. The trailhead is on the right just past a junction with FR 21, where you'll see a trailhead sign on the right. Turn right and follow the two-track road to where it ends at a gate.

Florida Trail:
Pat's Island to Hidden Pond

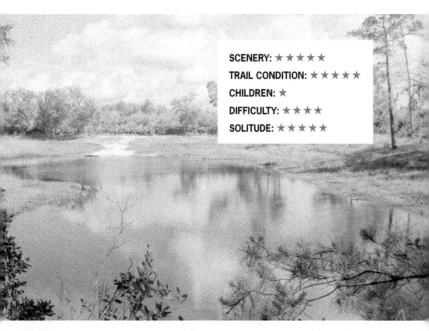

SCENERY: ★ ★ ★ ★ ★
TRAIL CONDITION: ★ ★ ★ ★ ★
CHILDREN: ★
DIFFICULTY: ★ ★ ★
SOLITUDE: ★ ★ ★ ★ ★

HIDDEN POND

GPS TRAILHEAD COORDINATES: N29° 15.443' W81 40.868'

DISTANCE & CONFIGURATION: 8.4-mile balloon

HIKING TIME: 3.5 hours

HIGHLIGHTS: Hidden Pond, panoramic views from ridges, Pat's Island historic site

ACCESS: Open 24/7. Free.

MAPS: USGS *Salt Springs*, Florida Trail Association

FACILITIES: None

WHEELCHAIR ACCESS: None

COMMENTS: Leashed dogs welcome. Primitive camping permitted. Foot traffic only. This is a desertlike area; bring plenty of water and use sun protection. Consult the prescribed fire map on the forest website before entering the area. Please do not disturb archaeological sites.

CONTACTS: Ocala National Forest: 352-236-0288; **www.fs.usda.gov/ocala.** Florida Trail Association: 352-378-8823; **floridatrail.org.**

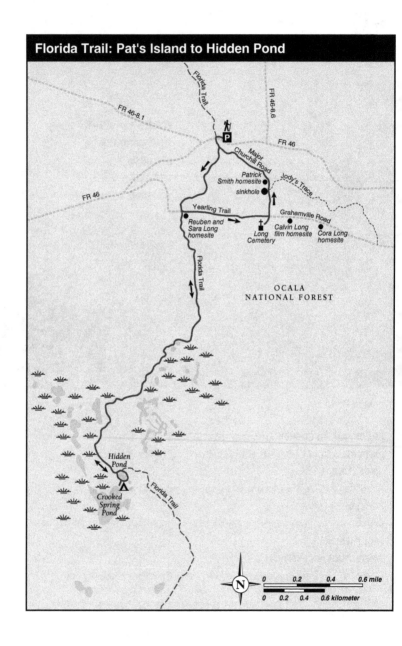

Florida Trail: Pat's Island to Hidden Pond

FR 46-8.1

Florida Trail

FR 46-8.6

FR 46

Major Churchill Road

Jody's Trace

Patrick Smith homesite

sinkhole

FR 46

Yearling Trail

Grahamville Road

Reuben and Sara Long homesite

Long Cemetery

Calvin Long film homesite

Cora Long homesite

Florida Trail

OCALA NATIONAL FOREST

Hidden Pond

Florida Trail

Crooked Spring Pond

N

| 0 | 0.2 | 0.4 | 0.6 mile |

| 0 | 0.2 | 0.4 | 0.6 kilometer |

Overview

One of the most popular hikes on the Florida Trail is also one of the most interesting. Hidden Pond is an oasis in the middle of the Juniper Prairie Wilderness, a designated wilderness area in the Ocala National Forest, and it lies nearly halfway between the two access points to the wilderness area—Juniper Springs (Hike 23) and Pat's Island. Pat's Island, in turn, has its own fascinating history to explore along the Yearling Trail, which this route also follows in part on the return trip.

Route Details

From the trailhead parking area, follow the narrow path west to where it emerges at some posts along the road. The connector trail turns right, but you can turn left and cross FR 46 to walk up to the Florida Trail crossing. Just beyond the road is a large JUNIPER PRAIRIE WILDERNESS sign. Heading south past it, you see tall longleaf pines in the distance. These signal the edge of Pat's Island, an island of longleaf pine amid the surrounding sea of the Big Scrub, the world's largest sand pine scrub forest. Passing a trail junction at a double-blazed post—part of the Yearling Trail, which you'll explore on the return trip—continue straight ahead.

Sand pine scrub is a very flammable habitat; in fact, it requires fire to properly regenerate. The USDA Forest Service has a no-fire-fighting policy in this wilderness area, which means when fires sweep through, they level everything. Major fires in 2007 and 2009 consumed the area, which is why you'll see many standing dead pine trunks and blacked oaks along this hike. Treat the ones near the trail as very real hazards, since they will fall across the footpath at some point.

Climbing uphill, where roots act as natural water bars in the footpath, you see signs of life. Nature heals quickly in this habitat, so the understory growth is extremely dense, and many of the surviving sand live oaks are lush with leaves again. Climbing up and down several ridges, you see tall, unscathed pines with open, grassy spots beneath them. Each of these ridges is an ancient sand dune, one of the rare places in Florida that the sea didn't cover, which is why the assemblage of plants in the Big Scrub includes many unusual species. Reaching an oak-shaded ridgetop, you find the second junction with the Yearling Trail at 0.8 mile. Continue straight ahead, following the Florida Trail as it descends to the first of many prairies in the Juniper Prairie Wilderness.

Climbing up and over the next ancient dune, you descend into a cluster of young sand pines and walk around the western edge of a larger prairie. The scrub forest along the next few miles of trail is the perfect height for Florida scrub-jay habitat. These jays are only found in Florida and only in the scrub; the Ocala National Forest has the highest concentration of them. We heard and saw dozens during this hike.

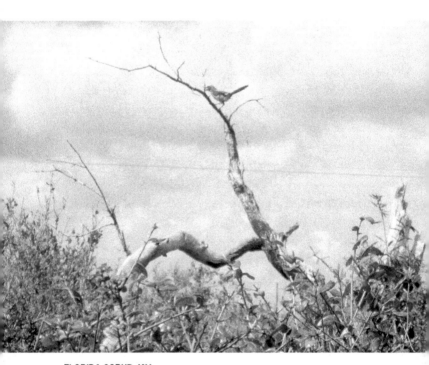

FLORIDA SCRUB-JAY

Rounding a swale, the trail climbs up to high ground from which you can survey more distant ridges and continues its journey toward that line of pines you see to the southeast. By 1.7 miles you're in a maturing sand pine forest. Most of the hiking through the Big Scrub is through soft sand, very much like beach sand, and can become tiresome after many hours of walking. The optimal time to visit is after a soaking rain, as the sand remains firm until it fully dries out.

Reaching an oak hammock, enjoy a moment of shade before the trail starts following the rim of a very large prairie. After climbing a hill, it circles a pond inside a sinkhole. From this bluff, you can see another prairie in the distance. Descending to the next prairie's edge, you can see a deep pond, covered in water lilies, that persists even when water levels are extremely low. Over the next rise, a similar pond is visible in another part of this prairie.

By 2.3 miles you finally reach that line of pines that you kept seeing in the distance since the second intersection with the Yearling Trail. The trail stays to the west of two prairies ringed by slash pines, climbing over the next ridge. Reaching the edge of the next prairie, you find the oak hammock blackened and dead from fire. Past the next pond is a live and vibrant oak hammock providing shade. Emerging onto the shore of another broad prairie, you pass large prickly pear cactus as the path climbs into the diminutive scrub. A high point provides a sweeping vista of prairies off to the horizon. As the trail begins to descend, you see your destination, Hidden Pond, at 3.6 miles.

Spring-fed Hidden Pond is tucked in a swale between the sand ridges, a basin of cool, clear water. One of the most popular destinations in Florida for an overnight backpacking trip—which means it's very busy on weekends—it's also one of the more picturesque spots along the Florida Trail. The orange blazes continue to the left and ascend the ridge past the pond, but this is your turnaround point. Step off the Florida Trail to walk around the pond clockwise; a footpath circles its rim. You'll enjoy several different perspectives on the pond as the trail climbs up into the oak hammock and leads you around to the camping area, simply flat, cleared spots under the oaks.

A prairie is on the other side of this ridge, and the gradient between pond and prairie means it's always breezy here, like a natural swamp cooler. The logs make a nice place for a midhike break. While you're snacking, listen for the chatter of scrub-jays, as a family lives in the oaks along the pond.

Leaving the camping area, complete your full circle around Hidden Pond until you're back to the Florida Trail. Juniper Springs is to the south, and Pat's Island is to the north. Turn left to start the return trip to Pat's Island. As you climb away from the pond, be sure you're headed northwest. At the top of this first ridge, you can see several ridges in quick succession ahead of you and two more in the far distance to your left. By 4.2 miles the trail drops out of the scrub forest to face charred trees along the prairie rim. Keep alert for an old trail going up to the right. Although it's the broader path, it's covered with logs to discourage its use. The Florida Trail stays close to the prairie rim, an obvious footpath snaking between the dead trees.

Climbing up and over the ridges, you pass the pine-rimmed prairies and return to the large prairie system with its deep ponds. At 5.5 miles, it almost looks like the trail plunges straight ahead and down into the sinkhole; make sure you take the sharp left here to stay on the bluffs above it. A mile later, after circling several more prairies, you ascend steeply to the shady intersection with the Yearling Trail. Going straight ahead saves almost a mile, but it's worth the extra footsteps to learn a little about pioneer life in the Big Scrub. Turn right.

Blazed with yellow blazes, the Yearling Trail leads you into the heart of Pat's Island, a historic settlement in the Big Scrub. In the 1840s, Patrick Smith, for whom the island was named, ran the post office. A circuit preacher from Paisley would arrive once a month to preach at the Chapel Methodist Church. At least a dozen families settled here, including Reuben and Sara Jane Long, who arrived in the fall of 1876. It was truly Florida's frontier, where growing sugar cane, corn, peas, beans, and watermelon, the Longs scraped out a life in a very harsh environment. When their young son Melvin found a fawn, they allowed him to raise it. Decades later, Melvin's brother

Calvin entertained Marjorie Kinnan Rawlings for a few days in 1938 and shared the family's stories, inspiring *The Yearling,* her Pulitzer Prize–winning novel.

When this trail was established, an interpretive map keyed to numbers on posts helped explain the significance of sites along the loop. Some of the original numbers and sites are now gone. The new map does not reflect all of the markers found along this loop. Marker 8 calls attention to a rainwater cistern, all that remains of the original Reuben Long homestead. Beyond it, the trail drops downhill into a bowl of slash pines, a prime location for fall wildflower viewing. As you walk past a row of young longleaf pines, notice how the trail has widened. You're on the Old Grahamville Road, a historic wagon road connecting the original settlements of the Big Scrub. The trail descends, reaching a junction at 7.4 miles.

Turn right at this junction to see the Long family cemetery. It's a quiet spot on the hill, still tended, with the tombstones of Reuben and Sara Jane showing their age. Return to the trail junction and continue straight through it. The broad path through the pines passes large sand live oaks with gnarled branches and a pine catfaced for turpentine tapping. Entering an oak hammock, you emerge along the rim of an enormous sinkhole. This is where the families of Pat's Island collected their water, in catch basins below sheets of limestone where tiny springs once dripped. To supplement this source, they used rainwater cisterns, and if the need arose, took a 4-mile round-trip to Silver Glen Springs for buckets of spring water.

This clearing is also the intersection with Jody's Trace, a trail that heads east to join the wagon trail and eventually reach the Yearling Trail Trailhead along FL 19. To stay on the loop around Pat's Island, continue past the sinkhole, to the left of Jody's Trace. Passing marker 5—where Patrick Smith's homestead was located—you reach marker 6, the Major Churchill Road. Keep to the right, leaving the leafy shade of Pat's Island for the scrub again. Look for gopher tortoise burrows along this stretch. By 8.2 miles you reach the trail junction with the Florida Trail. Turn right. After you pass the back side of the JUNIPER PRAIRIE WILDERNESS sign, cross the forest road toward the short posts to the right. Turn right to follow the path back to the Pat's Island Trailhead, wrapping up this 8.4-mile hike.

Nearby Attractions

Canoe and hike at Silver Glen Springs, one of the prettiest springs for swimming: **bit.ly/silverglensprings.** The takeout for Juniper Run is just up the road. To paddle through the Juniper Prairie Wilderness or relax under the oaks at the Juniper Springs Campground, head for Juniper Springs Recreation Area, where Hike 23 connects the springs: **bit.ly/juniperspringsrecarea.**

Directions

From the intersection of FL 40 and FL 19 in the Ocala National Forest (34 miles west of I-95 and 37 miles east of I-75), drive north 6.2 miles, passing the Juniper Wayside and then a few miles later, the entrances to Silver Glen Springs and the Yearling Trail. You'll see a PAT'S ISLAND TRAILHEAD sign directing you to the left onto FR 46. Follow this single-lane forest road (it's a little rugged but passable by passenger vehicles) for 2 miles. A sign directs you into the trailhead on the right.

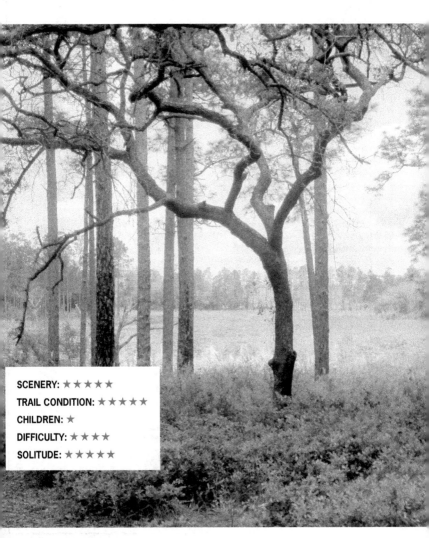

SCENERY: ★ ★ ★ ★ ★
TRAIL CONDITION: ★ ★ ★ ★ ★
CHILDREN: ★
DIFFICULTY: ★ ★ ★
SOLITUDE: ★ ★ ★ ★ ★

PENNER POND

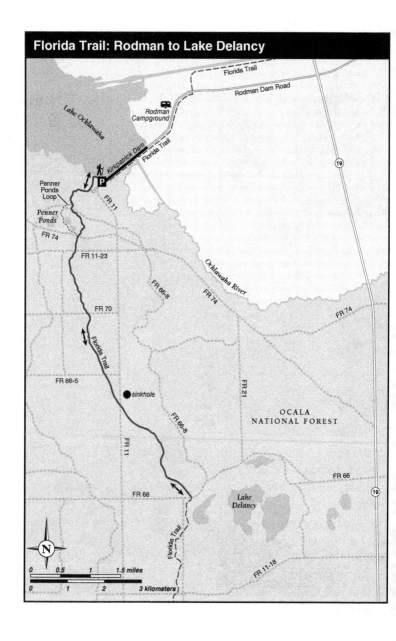

Florida Trail: Rodman to Lake Delancy

GPS TRAILHEAD COORDINATES: N29° 30.138' W81° 48.845'

DISTANCE & CONFIGURATION: 7-mile point to point

HIKING TIME: 3.5 hours

HIGHLIGHTS: Immersion in longleaf pine forest, abundant wildflowers, Rodman Reservoir views

ACCESS: Open 24/7. Free.

MAPS: USGS *Rodman*, Florida Trail Association

FACILITIES: Vault toilets are available at the Rodman Trailhead, with flush toilets and potable water available at far end of dam in a recreation area. Camping and toilets available at Delancy West Recreation Area November–April.

WHEELCHAIR ACCESS: None

COMMENTS: Leashed dogs welcome. Primitive camping permitted. Foot traffic only. No surface water exists south of Penner Ponds; bring plenty of water. Consult the prescribed fire map on the forest website before entering the area. Please do not disturb archaeological sites.

CONTACTS: Ocala National Forest: 352-236-0288; **www.fs.usda.gov/ocala.** Florida Trail Association: 352-378-8823; **floridatrail.org.**

Overview

One of the best hikes in Florida for immersion in the natural beauty of a longleaf pine forest, the Florida Trail between Rodman and Lake Delancy spends much of its time traversing Riverside Island, an island of longleaf pine spanning more than 9,200 acres within the larger Big Scrub ecosystem. Vast forests of longleaf once blanketed the Southeast from Virginia to Texas but were the first to fall to the logger's axe. Scarcely 2% of the original longleaf pine forests of America remain. With hilly terrain topped with this rare and special forest, this is a truly spectacular hike.

Route Details

Using two vehicles, this linear hike is a 7-mile walk between trail-heads. With one vehicle, we recommend you start at the Rodman Trailhead and walk south as far as you like; for the best immersion in the longleaf pine forest, go as far south as the sinkhole just beyond Forest Road 11 before turning around for a round-trip of 9 miles.

From the Rodman Trailhead, walk back toward the dam and make a left into the grassy, open area just before you reach Rodman Reservoir. As you pass an abandoned kiosk, you'll see orange blazes leading into the forest along the shore of this man-made lake. Spanish moss hangs in thick draperies from the live oaks, swaying in the breeze. The shore of the lake is choked with logs, which pop up from the lake bottom. In the 1960s, the Army Corps of Engineers used an enormous machine called a crusher-crawler to flatten the floodplain forest of the Ocklawaha River as part of their effort to build the Cross Florida Barge Canal. When the project was finally stopped in 1971, what remained was the reservoir, the dam, and one completed canal segment to a lock to the St. Johns River to the east. The struggle continues between state politicians, local residents, environmental groups, and government agencies as to the future of the reservoir and river valley. Meanwhile, there are several beautiful camping spots along the trail beneath the oaks.

By a quarter mile, the trail turns away from the water's edge and begins its journey into the Big Scrub through picturesque stands of oak hammock, the canopy of sand live oaks and rusty lyonia just a few feet above your head. The trail feels like a tunnel through this scrubby corridor, emerging at times into patches of sand pine scrub with taller pines before diving into the deeply shaded oak hammocks. Shield lichen, ball moss, and old man's beard dangle from the wizened trunks of these small trees. At 0.8 mile you reach a T intersection with the upper junction of the Penner Pond Trail, which is blue-blazed. Turn left to stay on the Florida Trail, tunneling through the scrub before crossing through a deep curve of soft sand on one of the official ATV trails.

As the forest canopy opens up to the right, you catch a glimpse of water lilies blooming on the surface of a flatwoods pond. Crossing an old blocked-off forest road, you can see more wetlands to the right. The trail climbs up into sandhills past a swale that cradles an ephemeral pond. Looping around a small stand of sand pine, the trail twists and curves through sandhill habitat, interwoven with patches of scrub.

At 1.7 miles the trail meets the lower junction of the Penner Pond Trail. The blue blazes lead downhill to the right toward one of the larger lily-dotted ponds. Continue straight ahead, crossing FR 74 to continue through a tunnel of scrub. An old wooden sign says Lake Delancy is 6 miles ahead, but it overstates the distance. Passing under a power line, the trail climbs up out of the scrub and into the rolling sandhills. You've reached Riverside Island. A vast, open understory is characteristic of the longleaf pine forest here. You'll see some trees with white bands, marked to indicate them as nesting trees for red-cockaded woodpeckers, who prefer trees a century old or more. By 2.5 miles you leave the longleaf briefly to walk into scrub, passing by some large prickly pear cacti in clearings on both sides of the trail. Emerging from the scrub to a swale of longleaf pine forest, the trail ascends through an expansive landscape of longleaf pine. This is hilly terrain on a large scale; you'll climb up and down hills for most of the rest of the hike. At 3.1 miles there is a marker 31 for a forest road crossing, at a stand of laurel oak. Sandhills and scrub intermingle along this portion of the trail.

As you enter the longleaf forest again, the change of habitat is dramatic. Crossing an unmarked forest road at 4.2 miles, the trail continues uphill through a vast landscape of rolling hills, the open understory enabling you to see the forest drop off to the horizon in every direction. There are only a few important ingredients that make up this very special habitat: the longleaf pines, most of them well on in years; turkey oaks, which in spring sport light green leaves; and wiregrass, the showy, soft taupe haze that covers the forest floor. On open patches of sand, you'll see prickly pear cactus and gopher apple, and amid the wiregrass, delicate wildflowers bloom.

Passing a dry sinkhole in the middle of the longleaf pine forest, the trail descends a long slope to FR 11, a major road through the Ocala National Forest. After you cross it at 4.5 miles, the trail enters a shady hammock of older live oaks clustered around a large sinkhole with an ephemeral pond inside it. This is a good, recognizable turnaround point if you're hiking out and back from the Rodman Trailhead.

Circling around the sinkhole through this beauty spot, you step right through a carved-out section of a fallen limb from one of the massive live oak trees. The red blooms of coral bean peep out of the understory in spring. Climbing away from the sinkhole, wiregrass yields to a mix of grasses under the pines that provides a bonanza of wildflowers. In springtime look for clusters of wooly pawpaw, with their draping ivory blooms; delicate roserush, a flower with serrated edges that almost looks like it floats on air, the stem is so slender; and green-eyes, low-growing yellow blossoms with a dark green "eye" in the center. Butterflies love the terrible thistle, with its purple flowers on tall stalks, and you'll see the delicate pink blooms of milkweed amid leaves sprawled against the forest floor.

At 5.3 miles you cross the indentation of a singletrack road, where a post marks the trail, and the longleaf forest around you stretches as far as the eye can see. Still surrounded by the longleaf forest, the trail enters a small hammock of sand live oaks, a spot in deeper shade. Beyond it, the landscape drops off to the left around a large, dry sinkhole. Passing a blaze on a post at an unmarked road, the trail continues straight ahead through the longleaf. The faintest trace of an old road cuts through the forest at 5.9 miles as the trail enters the shade of a stand of sand live oaks overlooking the next rolling ridge of longleaf pine. You spot some coontie—a native cycad—on the left as the trail descends into a bowl of sandhills, where turkey oaks outnumber the longleaf pines. Native yucca, or Adam's needle, seems well suited to this habitat, as it grows profusely here.

Passing a blaze on a thick post, where the trail seems like it goes right but turns left, you continue through the sandhills, where laurel oaks are scattered amid the turkey oaks and patches of prickly pear cactus. Walking through a hammock of tall, thin oaks with wiggly trunks, you can see the forest road to the right. At 6.9 miles you reach the edge of FR 66 and the entrance to Delancy West Recreation Area. If you parked inside the recreation area, walk across the road and through the entrance to end your hike after 7 miles.

Nearby Attractions

Camp just up the road at Rodman Campground for access to trails in this area: **bit.ly/rodmancampground.** Camp, hike, swim, paddle, and explore the Bear Swamp Trail at Salt Springs, a gem first written about by William Bartram in 1774: **bit.ly/saltspringsrec.** Ocklawaha Canoe Outpost can assist with rentals and shuttles for paddling the Ocklawaha River in this area and has campsites and cabins on the river: **outpostresort.com.** Hike 20, Davenport Landing Trail, can be accessed via FR 11 south to FR 77, the first turnoff on the left, although the road can get rough at times.

Directions

Rodman Trailhead: From the intersection of US 19 and CR 316 in Salt Springs, drive north along US 19 for 12.3 miles. Turn left onto the George Kirkpatrick Dam Road and drive 4.5 miles to the Rodman Trailhead on the far side of the dam, where the pavement ends. Please note that the dam crossing is closed every Wednesday from 8:30 a.m.–2 p.m. for maintenance. The trailhead can also be accessed via FR 11, a well-maintained, wide dirt road, by driving 9.6 miles north on FR 11 from CR 316 west of Salt Springs.

Delancy West Trailhead: From Rodman Trailhead, drive south on FR 11. After 5 miles you'll reach the junction with FR 66, where a sign should point the way to Delancy West Recreation Area. Turn left and drive east 1.1 miles to the recreation area. Delancy West is closed May–September, but you can park along FR 66 on the grassy shoulder near the trail crossing. Access is also available to Delancy West via FR 66 from US 19, but the 2.5-mile drive is much more difficult for a passenger vehicle due to deep washouts in the road.

23 # Juniper Springs Nature Trail

SCENERY: ★ ★ ★ ★ ★
TRAIL CONDITION: ★ ★ ★ ★ ★
CHILDREN: ★ ★ ★ ★ ★
DIFFICULTY: ★
SOLITUDE: ★ ★ ★

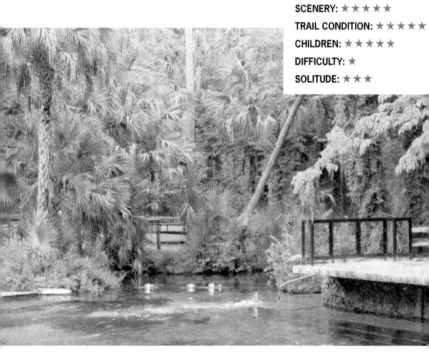

JUNIPER SPRINGS SWIMMING AREA

GPS TRAILHEAD COORDINATES: N29° 10.967' W81° 42.773'

DISTANCE & CONFIGURATION: 1.4-mile out-and-back

HIKING TIME: 1 hour

HIGHLIGHTS: Hidden Pond, panoramic views from ridges, Pat's Island historic site

ACCESS: Daily, 8 a.m.–8 p.m.; closing hours vary by season. Day-use fee: $5 per person; registered campers pay no additional entrance fee to visit the springs.

MAPS: USGS *Juniper Springs*, Ocala National Forest website

FACILITIES: Campground, concession stand/camp store, picnic areas, swimming area

WHEELCHAIR ACCESS: Fully accessible

COMMENTS: Leashed dogs welcome. The boardwalk is optimized for wheelchairs, with passing lanes in quite a few spots. Please stay on the boardwalk—it keeps visitors from trampling on the fragile banks of the two spring runs.

CONTACTS: Ocala National Forest: 352-236-0288; **www.fs.usda.gov/ocala**

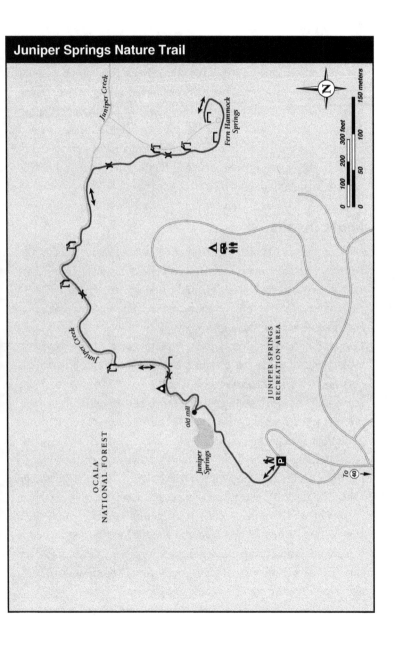

Overview

Nowhere else on Earth will you see the spectacle of nature found at the end of this short but beautiful boardwalk through an oasis of verdant green surrounding two very different spring basins. Developed into a recreation area in the 1930s by the Civilian Conservation Corps, Juniper Springs is a favorite for swimmers. At the other end of the trail, Fern Hammock Springs provides a mesmerizing collection of pulsating turquoise pools and frantic underwater sand boils you can stare into for hours.

Route Details

Walk up the paved path from the parking area, passing through the building with the concession stand and restrooms. Follow the Chattahoochee stone path along the right side of Juniper Springs as it circles around to the mill house, where the museum may be open. Interpretive panels share the story of the Civilian Conservation Corps at Juniper Springs. Leaving the mill, look for the NATURE TRAIL sign to point you toward a boardwalk with an observation deck for viewing the constant churn of the mill. You walk past an old stone arch bridge crumbling into the spring run. It's officially blocked off from use. Notice the crystalline clarity of the water as it pours out of Juniper Springs.

Although the name of the trail has always been the Juniper Springs Nature Trail, a new interpretive sign, "Welcome to Juniper Creek Nature Trail," greets you as you start down the trail, passing a spot where you can see paddlers at the put-in for Juniper Run. Just beyond the nature trail sign, look down to the left. The trees obscure a small collection of very pretty little spring boils. Small fish dart through them as they erupt from the bottom of the waterway, with white sand spilling out in constant tiny geysers.

Crossing a bridge with a low-hanging cabbage palm over it, the boardwalk turns left at a bench. Look for brown nature-trail signs along the boardwalk with interpretive information about plants.

Some of the signs, like the one by the needle palms, are quite over-sized, pulling your gaze away from the landscape.

At 0.3 mile you reach the first of the decks along the creek. You can see deeper water here where the waterway makes the bend, a crystal clear view straight to the bottom. Don't be surprised to see a kayaker or canoeist slip past; the 7-mile Juniper Run is one of the most popular paddling trails in the state. Swarms of ferns cover the forest floor, loving this humid habitat, with netted chain, cinnamon fern, and royal fern peeping out from under clusters of needle palms. You see a tipped-over oak as the trail curves to the right through an area with a very dense understory of blackberry bushes. A swath of canopy is missing, thanks to hurricane damage nearly a decade ago. Another cabbage palm leans in close to the boardwalk. Crossing a small bridge with the faintest trickle of a tributary flowing under it, you can still see the creek on the left.

At the next observation deck, watch the fish drift by. Here, you can tell the floodplain aspect of this waterway, the smoothness of the bottom and the sides from when water rushed through at a stronger rate of speed. Springs do ebb and flow over time. Sadly, there are major springs in Florida that were swimming holes a generation ago and are now dry because growing population density or industry nearby siphoned the water from the aquifer, choking off the spring. Being in the middle of the Ocala National Forest helps protect the springs here from that fate.

Resurrection fern renders the limbs of the live oaks overhead fuzzy and green. The boardwalk makes a sharp right after you leave the deck, moving away from the creek into a much denser oak hammock. Grapevines make an impassable, knotted tangle in most directions. At 0.5 mile take a left. There is another observation deck where you can watch the flow of Juniper Creek. Back on the main boardwalk, you pass a small staircase leading to a narrow path to the campground. Stay on the boardwalk. The canopy opens up again, showing off the larger live oaks and cabbage palms—and poison ivy, which flourishes through this part of the forest.

Shaded by palm fronds from young cabbage palms, the boardwalk loses a little elevation. The next observation deck is just a step off the main boardwalk, with a tiny bridge soon after. The boardwalk winds back and forth beneath the canopy of live oaks and cabbage palms. As you come to the fourth deck—the one with the pileated woodpecker interpretive sign—step over to the waterway and notice the change in direction. The tape grass is flattened by the strength of the outflow here and is going the opposite direction from what you've seen thus far. You're no longer along Juniper Run but following Fern Hammock Run, a tributary that feeds it.

Crossing the next bridge, you come to a grassy area with pines towering overhead. From a deck, you can see the flow of deeper water out of Fern Hammock Springs. At 0.7 mile the boardwalk ends at a T intersection and a sign, NATURE TRAIL CONCLUSION. RETURN TO SWIM SITE BY RETRACING TRAIL. However, the best is yet to come! Turn left to walk to Fern Hammock Springs, best visible from the bridge you see ahead.

From the bridge, if you look directly below you over the right side, you'll see a massive sand boil spring. In the crystalline water, it looks like a sandstorm when it's pumping. On the other side is the spring basin, impressive in its singular beauty. Nowhere else in the world have we found a spring as enchanting. It's impossible to swim here, given the constantly shifting sands of the basin and the wildlife, but nature puts on an incredible show. There are tiny bubblers and big boils, and a strange collection of turquoise and gray blobs that continually expand and contract like the paint pots of Yellowstone beneath the water's surface.

Cross the bridge and continue along the fence to circle around the spring and enjoy different perspectives on the basin. Trail's end is at a concrete bench facing the spring beyond pavilion 4, a CCC-era picnic shelter in disrepair. Sit and enjoy the show. Fish, turtles, and the occasional alligator drift just below the placid surface as if they were floating on air, ignoring nature's frenzy below them.

Turn around and retrace your steps across the bridge over Fern Hammock Springs. Turn right to rejoin the boardwalk, and follow it back to Juniper Springs. You'll start hearing the distinctive chug of the water wheel at the old mill by 1.2 miles. Take the path around the mill house and springs to the left, and walk through the bathhouse and concession area to exit. You reach the parking area after 1.4 miles.

Nearby Attractions

Juniper Springs Recreation Area is a hub for outdoor recreation, including one of the best paddling runs in the state; check at the concessionaire for rates and shuttle information: **bit.ly/junipersprings recarea.** The Florida Trail crosses the entrance road and continues north to Hidden Pond, the endpoint for Hike 21, Florida Trail: Pat's Island to Hidden Pond. Canoe and hike at Silver Glen Springs, one of the prettiest springs for swimming: **bit.ly/silverglensprings.**

Directions

From I-75, Exit 352, drive east on FL 40 through Ocala and Silver Springs and into the Ocala National Forest, reaching the entrance for Juniper Springs after 30 miles. From I-95, Exit 268, drive west on FL 40, crossing the St. Johns River at Astor, to reach the entrance to Juniper Springs after 38.5 miles. Follow the park road north to the day-use area.

24

Lake Eaton Trails

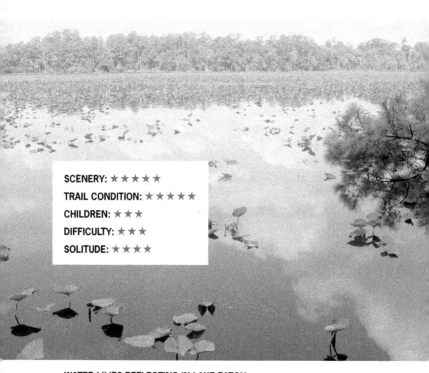

SCENERY: ★ ★ ★ ★ ★
TRAIL CONDITION: ★ ★ ★ ★ ★
CHILDREN: ★ ★ ★
DIFFICULTY: ★ ★ ★
SOLITUDE: ★ ★ ★ ★

WATER LILIES REFLECTING IN LAKE EATON

GPS TRAILHEAD COORDINATES: N29° 15.785' W81° 51.306'

DISTANCE & CONFIGURATION: 4.2-mile double loop

HIKING TIME: 2.5 hours

HIGHLIGHTS: Lake boardwalks, climbing in and out of the sinkhole

ACCESS: Open 24/7. Free.

MAPS: USGS *Lake Kerr*, Ocala National Forest website

FACILITIES: Kiosks and interpretive information, composting toilet, benches

WHEELCHAIR ACCESS: None

COMMENTS: Access roads are dirt and can be rough. This habitat is Florida's desert. Take plenty of water for your hike.

CONTACTS: Ocala National Forest: 352-236-0288; **www.fs.usda.gov/ocala**

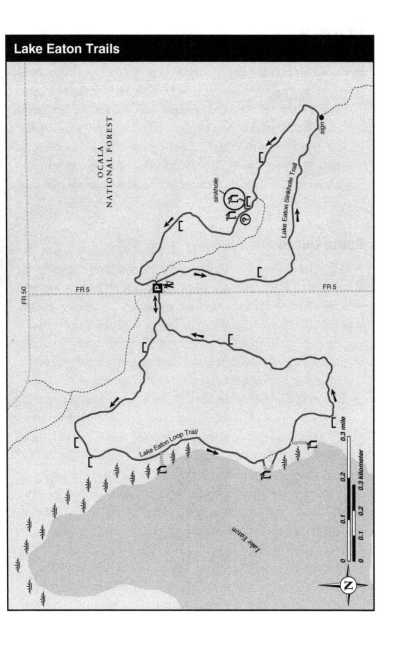

Lake Eaton Trails

OCALA NATIONAL FOREST

sinkhole

Lake Eaton Sinkhole Trail

FR 50

FR 5

FR 5

P

Lake Eaton Loop Trail

Lake Eaton

0   0.1   0.2   0.3 mile

0   0.1   0.2   0.3 kilometer

N

Overview

Introducing you to the heart of the Big Scrub—the desertlike habitat that the Ocala National Forest exists to protect—the Lake Eaton Trails showcase this high, dry ecosystem, along with two fascinating natural features. The Lake Eaton Sinkhole, more than 450 feet across and 80 feet deep, is a relatively young phenomenon compared to Lake Eaton itself, a large, ancient sinkhole lake. Both are karst features, formed by slightly acidic water flowing through limestone over eons. Beneath the bright white sands of the scrub, limestone bedrock holds the secrets of how water flows through this dry landscape—underground.

Route Details

Walk up to the Lake Eaton Sinkhole Trail entrance, near the restroom. Turn right to start the loop. You immediately come to a junction with the Shortcut Trail; continue straight ahead. Slipping behind the restroom, the trail starts snaking its way through the scrub forest. A high, dry habitat, scrub is Florida's desert. The plants around you have adapted to survive in sandy soil with little water to nourish them.

Popping out into the sun, you walk past a stand of tall sand pines nearing the end of their lives, about 70 years. Losing elevation, the trail winds past chopped-up logs. They speak to the amount of work that had to be done to reopen the trails of the Ocala National Forest after the hurricanes of the last decade. Myrtle oak and Chapman oak dominate the understory.

By a quarter mile, a young canopy of oaks shades the trail. You can hear songbirds in the trees. Keep alert for reptiles sunning themselves in the puddles of sunlight that punctuate this habitat. Beyond a large bench, you reach an old trail junction. Turn left to head down a shaded tunnel of diminutive oak scrub. Watch for scrub hickory, a tiny version of hickory with the leaf structure you'd expect, and scrub holly. Passing another stand of tall sand pine at 0.5 mile, the trail makes a sharp left. Just beyond a Florida rosemary bush, several species of lichen fill the crook of one small oak tree. Passing a trail marker, continue on the obvious trail—do not turn off to the right.

Beyond a bench, the twisting limbs of rusty lyonia shade the trail. After a slight downhill, you reach the Shortcut Trail. Pass this junction, with its cluster of interpretive signs, and continue downhill to meet the Lake Eaton Sinkhole. A staircase with several landings leads you down into its interior, reaching the lowest deck at 1.3 miles. With vegetation covering the slopes, there isn't much to see in the way of karst features; unlike Devil's Millhopper (Hike 4), water does not play an active role in shaping this formation. But water—or lack thereof—caused the ground to collapse, forming this hole that's more than 450 feet across and 80 feet deep. It's been here a long time, judging from the size of the trees that emerge from its bottom, forming its own microclimate. Climb back up the stairs and take the time to visit the kiosk at the overlook, as it provides a great deal of detail about how sinkholes happen.

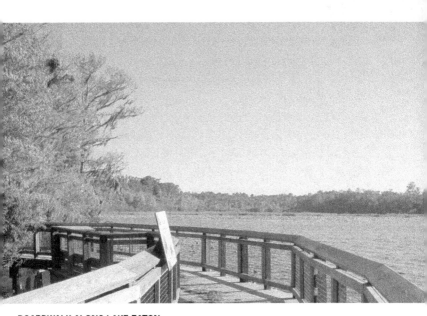

BOARDWALK ALONG LAKE EATON

A short set of steps leads uphill to the meandering path through the scrub. Florida rosemary thrives past the next interpretive marker, with some particularly tall specimens flanking the trail. After a denser oak scrub with young sand pines, the trail passes the next bench. It loses a little elevation at an interpretive sign on bears, reaching the end of the loop. Turn right to exit to the parking area. You've hiked 1.8 miles.

Look for the LAKE EATON TRAIL sign, and cross FR 5 to start the second loop, which leads you to the lake. At the kiosk, keep right and follow the trail downhill. This is a young scrub forest, with sand pines no more than 20 feet tall. It's the ideal habitat for the Florida scrub-jay, an endemic Florida bird seen throughout the Big Scrub of the Ocala National Forest. Past a large bench, you feel a definite downhill. Crossing an old jeep road, continue straight ahead.

Passing an interpretive sign, the trail continues downhill between the young sand pines, often compared to the Charlie Brown Christmas tree. Each December, the Ocala National Forest allows cutting of sand pines from a designated area. Look to the right and you can see how tightly the young sand pines and young oaks cluster together in this habitat. It takes a forest fire to thin them out. One prickly pear cactus is the centerpiece of a clearing lined with saw palmetto.

The trail makes a sharp turn as it passes the next bench, entering an older, more well-established oak forest. Another bench is near an old fencepost with a marker pointing straight ahead. Crispy with leaf litter, the footpath feels like an old, narrow wagon road under a canopy of oaks. When you see blue sky to the right, you're nearing the lake; the forest of tall slash pines and cabbage palms rustles in the breeze. At 2.6 miles you reach the first boardwalk to Lake Eaton. Turn right. The boardwalk ends at an observation deck with an unobstructed view of the cypress-lined lake, including the boat ramp and youth camp on the far shores. A large pine leans out gracefully over the water to the right.

Return along the boardwalk and make a right to continue the loop. Passing a sign for an old service road, continue straight ahead. At a sign that says PARKING, take the narrow trail to the right. It leads to the next boardwalk, which arcs out over the waters of Lake Eaton and back into the forest. Enjoy the sweeping view. Follow the footpath back to the main trail, reaching it at an interpretive sign. Turn right.

You come to the third and final boardwalk at 3.2 miles. The surface can be slippery, as pine needles and cones pile up on it. It leads to an observation deck over a cove in Lake Eaton, a nice place to watch for birds and wildlife from the bench.

Returning to the main trail, turn right. Passing a bench on the right, the trail turns left past a split rail fence to start the ascent back to the trailhead. As you climb back into the oak scrub, look for streamers of old man's beard hanging from the oaks and oddly shaped insect galls on the shiny lyonia. The footpath dips downhill briefly because of a sinkhole hidden in the dense forest. Passing another bench, it rises up into sand pine scrub, with an interpretive marker at 4 miles. As the sand gets softer underfoot, you see an interpretive sign on the ancient forest. Reaching the kiosk, turn right and continue to the trailhead, completing this 4.2-mile hike.

Nearby Attractions

Down a rough road, Lake Eaton Campground provides 14 beautiful seasonal sites along the lake: **bit.ly/camplakeeaton.** From the trailhead on NE 170th Avenue, follow the Florida Trail to Eaton Creek: **floridahikes.com/florida-trail-ocala.** At Forest Corners, Marie's Home Cookin is one of our favorites—don't miss their ice cream puff!

Directions

From I-75, Exit 352, follow FL 40 east through Ocala and Silver Springs 13.5 miles to Nuby's Corner, the first traffic light past the big bridge over the Ocklawaha River. Turn left on CR 314. Continue 8.6 miles. Just past CR 314A and a side road to the FWC Youth Camp, watch for FR 50 (NE 172nd Avenue Road) to the right. Follow this rough and bumpy dirt road 0.9 mile to a sign at FR 5, the first road on the right. Turn right and continue 0.2 mile to the parking area on the left.

25

Salt Springs Observation Trail

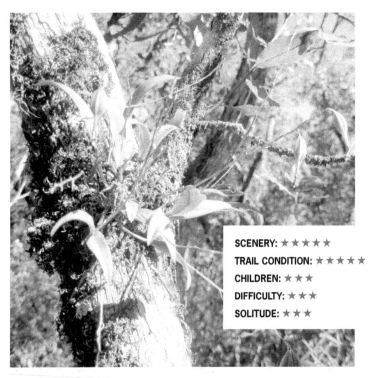

SCENERY: ★ ★ ★ ★ ★
TRAIL CONDITION: ★ ★ ★ ★ ★
CHILDREN: ★ ★ ★
DIFFICULTY: ★ ★ ★
SOLITUDE: ★ ★ ★

GREENFLY ORCHIDS WITH SEED PODS

GPS TRAILHEAD COORDINATES: N29° 20.414' W81° 43.740'

DISTANCE & CONFIGURATION: 2-mile balloon

HIKING TIME: 1 hour

HIGHLIGHTS: Picturesque scrub forest, excellent observation point

ACCESS: Open 24/7. Free.

MAPS: USGS *Salt Springs*, Ocala National Forest website

FACILITIES: Kiosks and interpretive information, benches

WHEELCHAIR ACCESS: None

COMMENTS: Leashed dogs welcome. Bicycles not permitted. Be alert to wildlife on and around this trail. On some signage, the trail is called the Salt Springs Loop Trail.

CONTACTS: Ocala National Forest: 352-236-0288; **www.fs.usda.gov/ocala**

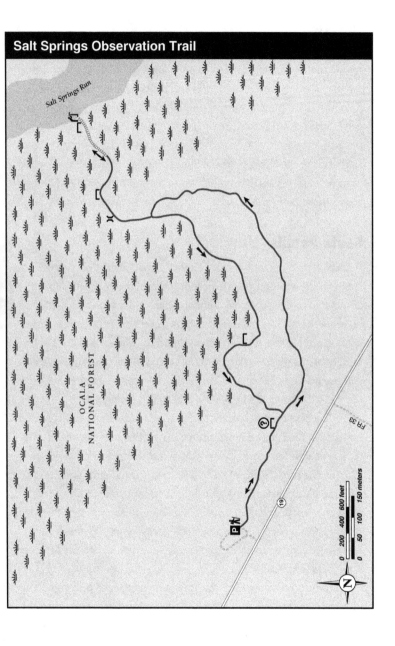

Salt Springs Observation Trail

Overview

When William Bartram paddled up Salt Springs Run in 1774, he found the untouched beauty of Salt Springs, "the waters of which are so extremely clear as to be absolutely diaphanous." As the springs flow past a simple platform at the bottom of this nature trail loop, you'll have the opportunity to observe not just the waters but also the teeming life within and around them. At one of the easiest to access trailheads in the Ocala National Forest, the Salt Springs Observation Trail provides a gentle introduction to several of the major habitats found throughout the forest.

Route Details

A detailed map on a kiosk at the parking area provides an overview of the loop. The well-defined trail descends through a younger scrub forest dominated by Chapman oak, sand live oak, and myrtle oak, with trees no more than 20 feet tall. A slash pine towers over the low canopy of scrub. Shield lichen blankets fallen branches, while red blanket lichen mimics blazes on the oak trunks. As you continue the gentle descent, you reach a large bench at 0.2 mile and, in just a few more footsteps, the trail junction at the top of the loop trail. Keep right.

The oak scrub here is more mature. Sand live oaks have gnarled limbs that form natural sculptures, to be matched by the slender but crooked branches of rusty lyonia, also known as crookedwood. Lichens and mosses carpet tree limbs, creating hanging gardens that, in some places, are graced with long, seafoam-colored streamers of old man's beard. Sphagnum moss and shiny blueberry mark the edge the trail. Coral bean pokes up from the forest floor in puddles of sunshine between the trees. In one sunny spot, you pass a prickly pear cactus that's at least 4 feet tall.

Continuing downhill, the trail tunnels deeper into the scrub forest, where the white blossoms of hammock snakeroot brighten the trail in fall and Southern magnolias drop their big leaves across the footpath. A keen observer will notice the Florida dogwood among them, only showy during its spring blooming season. Descending past American beautyberry that droops into the trail, you enter a forest of very small trees, spindly scrub oaks all crowded together with some sparkleberry among them. Amid more magnolias and dogwoods, the trail keeps up the steady drop in elevation, passing a large clump of saw palmetto.

The gnarled limbs of the sand live oaks are especially picturesque around a half mile, forming the canopy above. Carpeted with leaf litter, the trail continues a steady descent. Looking off to the right, you can see some tall sand pines in the distance, but for the most part the trail remains in a deeply shaded corridor of scrub oaks and rusty lyonia, twisting back and forth. As the trail begins to flatten out, you walk beneath another well-knit canopy of sand live oaks with lichens cradled in their branches. Passing between two split rail fences, where deer moss grows in copious quantity on the forest floor, the trail continues its subtle descent and the trees crowd in much more closely.

Reaching a T intersection with the other side of the loop, you see signs for the parking area and the boardwalk at 0.8 mile. Turn right. A linear passage flanked by deer moss, the trail descends slightly and narrows beneath the low canopy of oak scrub. Switch cane grows in a sometimes-soggy area near a small bridge where water trickles out of a bayhead. Cabbage palms, oaks, and pines tower above a substantial bench. To the left you see some open sky, outlining the location of Salt Springs Run. The footpath becomes a soft carpet of pine needles as you walk beneath the tall pines.

By 1 mile you reach a substantial boardwalk with tall rails on both sides. Chances are its surface will be covered in leaves, since no one rakes the leaves that the hickories, sweetgums, and red maples shower down each winter. You see standing water in puddles amid the cabbage palms in the floodplain. Royal fern and cinnamon fern thrive in these shady, wet spaces. Fronds smack you in the face as you make your way to the observation platform.

Plan to spend some time at the observation platform, as patience is rewarded along this pristine spring-fed waterway. During our visit, we watched a family of otters tumbling their way down one side of the run as a bald eagle circled numerous times. An alligator surveyed us from the cover of water spangles as coots nudged their way through dense vegetation. Turtles sunned on logs. Crystal clear water flows beneath the deck, although an array of dead aquatic plants chokes the near shore.

Return along the boardwalk and through the pine flatwoods to the trail intersection at the bottom of the loop, reaching it at 1.3 miles. Continue straight ahead to follow the other side of the loop back

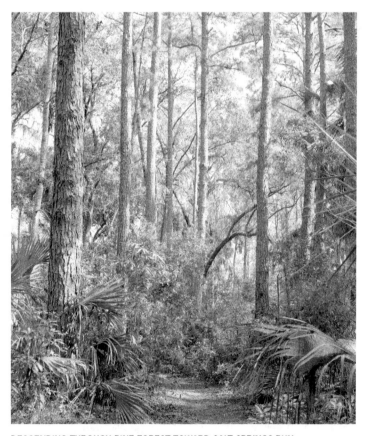

DESCENDING THROUGH PINE FOREST TOWARD SALT SPRINGS RUN

to the parking area. It starts out as a straightaway, with little shade, although slash pines tower overhead. Passing a split rail fence, the trail turns right and becomes shadier as it enters the oak scrub again. With a pine needle–cushioned path underfoot, it's a comfortable walk. As you ascend beneath a canopy of Southern magnolias, you start to hear the traffic on FL 19. Several pieces of split rail fence guide you in the right direction. The trail curves right, reaching another sturdy bench.

Entering a corridor of sunshine framed by saw palmetto, the trail zigzags for a short stretch. Although the climb has been gentle, as the trail draws closer to the loop junction, it suddenly ascends more steeply. By 1.8 miles you complete the loop. Turn right to exit. Walking back uphill to the parking area, you end your hike near the kiosk after 2 miles.

Nearby Attractions

Swim in the crystalline source of the waterway you just visited at Salt Springs Recreation Area: **bit.ly/saltspringsrec.** Or paddle down Salt Springs Run with a rental at the Salt Springs Marina: **bit.ly/saltsprings marina.** Oversized lunch specials are the norm at our local haunt, the Square Meal: **bit.ly/squaremealsaltspgs.**

Directions

From I-75, Exit 352, follow FL 40 east through Ocala and Silver Springs for 13.5 miles to Nuby's Corner, the first traffic light past the big bridge over the Ocklawaha River. Turn left on CR 314. Continue 18 miles to Salt Springs, where CR 314 ends at FL 19. Turn right and drive 0.7 mile to the trailhead entrance on the left, marked by a large sign.

Cross Florida Greenway (Hikes 26–30)

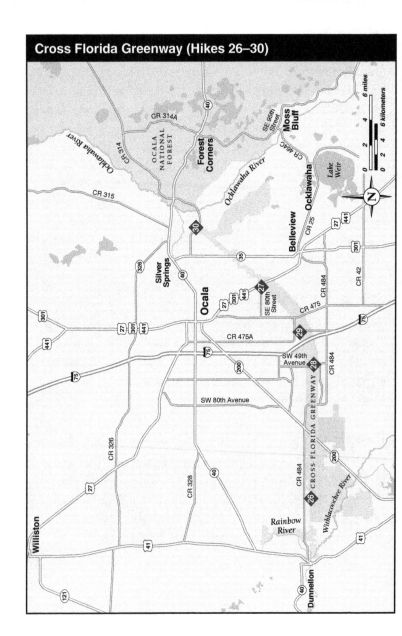

Cross Florida Greenway

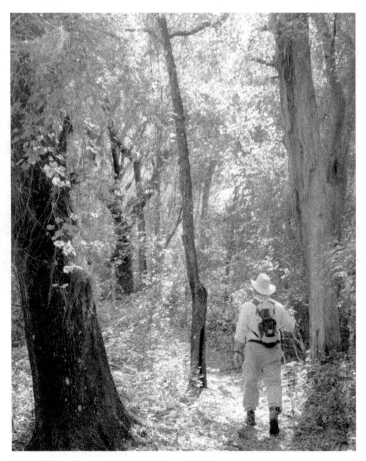

HIKING AT SANTOS; *see Hike 27, page 186*

26

Florida Trail: Pruitt

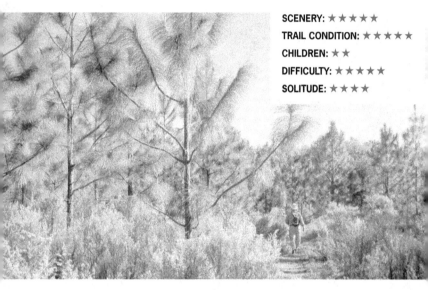

SCENERY: ★ ★ ★ ★ ★
TRAIL CONDITION: ★ ★ ★ ★
CHILDREN: ★ ★
DIFFICULTY: ★ ★ ★ ★ ★
SOLITUDE: ★ ★ ★

HIKING THROUGH A RESTORED LONGLEAF PINE FOREST

GPS TRAILHEAD COORDINATES: N29° 02.732' W82° 22.662'

DISTANCE & CONFIGURATION: 10.4-mile out-and-back

HIKING TIME: 4.5 hours

HIGHLIGHTS: Ancient oak trees, rugged terrain with switchbacks, canal views

ACCESS: Daily, sunrise–sunset; open for backpacking 24/7. Free.

MAPS: USGS *Dunnellon*

FACILITIES: Portable toilet and water fountain at trailhead, benches along trail

WHEELCHAIR ACCESS: None

COMMENTS: Leashed dogs welcome. Backpackers may camp along the trail with a free permit; call the Sharpes Ferry Office. No permit required for Florida Trail Association members.

Normally, it would also be possible to hike from the Pruitt Trailhead to the Ross Prairie Trailhead, a 6-mile linear walk; however, the Florida Department of Transportation is in the process of widening FL 200. This makes a traverse through the construction zone (if at all possible), even less safe than scurrying across the high-speed-traffic highway to the trailhead. The good news: When construction is done, there will be an underpass for recreational users and wildlife.

CONTACTS: Office of Greenways and Trails, Sharpes Ferry Office: 352-236-7143; **floridahikes.com/florida-trail-cross-florida-greenway.** Florida Trail Association: 352-378-8823; **floridatrail.org.**

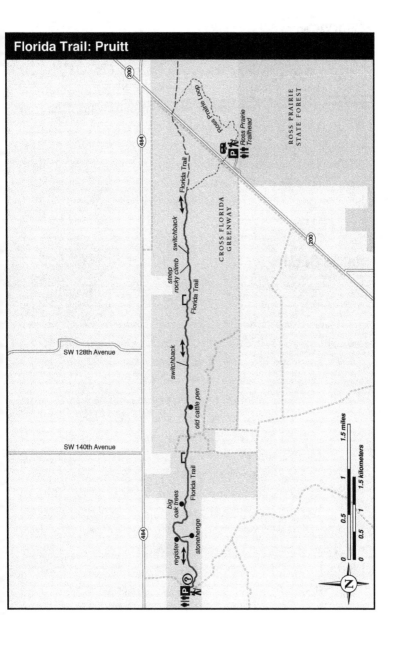

Florida Trail: Pruitt

Overview

It's not just the ancient live oaks but also the switchbacks and scrambles, the habitat diversity, the stories that the landscape tells, and "Stonehenge." These are some of the reasons that the Pruitt section of the Florida Trail, the westernmost portion of the trail on the Cross Florida Greenway, is one of my favorite hikes in the region. Granted, we might be biased, since Sandra maintained this section of the Florida Trail for quite a few years, but once you've hiked it, you'll understand why it calls you back again and again. On a rugged out-and-back hike of 10.4 miles, you'll see how native habitats swarmed back over a miles-long man-made gash in the earth and reclaimed the land.

Route Details

Starting at the trail kiosk and FLORIDA TRAIL sign, follow the limerock road—which is also the equestrian trail—into an open prairie. Blazes are infrequent. As the road curves to the left, look to the right for a sign in the distance. It marks a trailhead for adjacent Halpata Tastanaki Preserve, which serves as a stopover point for the juvenile whooping cranes of Operation Migration each season on their flight south. Although this vast prairie is rarely wet, there are indicator plants—black needlerush, wax myrtle, Virginia willow—that say it could flood, and indeed it has, which is why the Florida Trail follows the road.

At 0.6 mile you reach the corner of a fence. It is here at a FLORIDA TRAIL sign that the footpath begins in earnest, turning left off the road to head for the cool shade of a live oak hammock. Reaching a large FLORIDA TRAIL sign under the oaks, you'll see a trail register just beyond. Take the side trail to the right to see "Stonehenge," a circle of limestone boulders that form the Pruitt Memorial.

After signing the trail register, continue walking beneath the ancient oaks. The trail pops out into the sun to cross a scrubby spot en route to the next oak hammock, where resurrection fern grows not just on the limbs overhead but on the tree trunks and roots, too.

Birdsong fills the air as the trail follows a corridor of oaks flanked by prairie. By 1.2 miles you reach a grove of particularly large live oaks. The first one on the left is so large it could take six people to reach around it. Many of the trees have limbs as thick as a normal tree trunk that arch overhead to create a dense canopy. The next oak hammock, split by an old forest road, also has trees of spectacular size. Beyond it, the trail curves left to skirt an arm of the prairie. As you cross a sand road, you see a kiosk to the right for the equestrian trail system. Then it's up, up, and up!

When the switchback levels out, the trail is now atop a levee created by dirt piled here during construction of the Cross Florida Barge Canal in 1936. The forest floor undulates, in part from erosion, in part from hog damage. Be careful not to trip on roots. The perspective here is almost like a canopy walk, as you can look out into the live oak canopy on both sides of the levee. Ferns, fungi, and orchids are at eye level. Although the forest on top of the levee can be no more than 75 years old, it's amazing to see the size of the loblolly pines and cedars growing here. Looking down to the right, you can see the equestrian trail and an open prairie inside the bottom of the former canal route. The levee drops off precipitously on the left.

At 1.8 miles the trail turns left and goes down that steep slope, passing a lone cabbage palm before it makes a sharp right to go through a cluster of sand live oaks. The understory is crowded with young oaks, which yield to a grove of ancient live oaks draped in Spanish moss. Crossing the equestrian trail, you pass a bench and head into a meadow of planted longleaf pines. Beyond the pines, the trail leads you beneath more ancient oaks. Crossing a firebreak, you enter a laurel oak forest, the climax forest of the sandhill habitat, where the trees are about the same age as the canal diggings and at the end of their life span. The forest floor is littered with fallen logs covered in swarms of fungi.

Transitioning into an oak scrub with an open, parklike understory, the trail is surrounded by sand live oaks and lichens emerging from the white sand. As the footpath gains a little elevation, you rise up into the sandhills. Wiregrass covers the forest floor beneath the longleaf pines and turkey oaks. A big Florida rosemary shrub stands out alone in a patch of relict scrub. Crossing a firebreak at 2.6 miles, an old wooden cattle pen is visible to the right. In the years between the end of canal building here and the conversion of the land for recreational uses (1998), ranchers held cattle leases on this land.

The trail makes a full frontal assault on the next levee. There are nice views down into the forest on both sides, and a number of limestone boulders atop this hill. The natural-looking ravines are covered in leaves and duff. Between the cabbage palms sprouting from the levee and the limestone boulders, it looks like a tropical karst landscape from the Caribbean. The ravines are deeply cut, with steep drop-offs everywhere. You descend off this second levee under the cover of sand live oaks, crossing a limerock road at 3.1 miles.

Entering a rolling sandhill habitat, you see longleaf pines here in their various stages of life. Some look like the wiregrass that surrounds them, and others are shaped like bottlebrushes or saguaro cactus. Above them all are towering giants dropping giant pinecones on the forest floor. Crossing an old trail, you walk through a thicket of shoulder-height oaks that crowd right up to the footpath.

On the far side of a two-track jeep road, the trail ascends up a curving switchback. Limestone boulders, some painted with orange blazes, are scattered everywhere, poking out of the leaf litter beneath the oaks and pines. Reaching a bench at 3.8 miles, the trail turns right and drops steeply downhill to a lower terrace. It's the finest place along the Cross Florida Greenway for a close-up look at what the canal was going to look like.

If you examine a topographical map of this area, you'll see a series of disconnected rectangular lakes. This is the most prominent one. There is a "gator hole" pond in its bottom, down a beaten path, but we've also seen this canal basin brimming with water after a hurricane's worth of rain. Most of the time, all that grows in the basin is wax myrtle and Virginia willow, dog fennel and grasses. The footpath winds back and forth on the rim of the terrace, providing scenic views.

The trail veers left to ascend steeply to the top of the levee, only to descend again down a tall switchback at 4.4 miles. Crossing a sand road, it passes through a laurel oak forest, with islands of scrub and sandhill. Crossing the road a second time, the trail ascends into the naturally rolling landscape of the sandhills, its tall longleaf pines and turkey oaks resplendent in fall color. Just past a firebreak, the pine needles are especially thick underfoot, cradled in a natural bowl in the landscape. Climbing uphill from this bowl, you reach the turnaround point for this hike: the junction of the Florida Trail and the Ross Prairie Loop at a bench at 5.2 miles. There is a trail register here to sign.

It's only 0.8 mile to the Ross Prairie Trailhead, and 1.2 miles along the Florida Trail to FL 200. However, because of a road-widening project on FL 200, it's neither advisable (and, at times, will be impossible) to park a car on the shoulder or to cross the road at either location. The good news is that when the road project is complete, there will be an underpass for hikers on the Ross Prairie Loop. Meanwhile, it's best to turn around here after you take a break and hydrate. Return along the orange blazes to the Pruitt Trailhead for a 10.4-mile round-trip, enjoying the peace and solitude of this unique section of trail.

Nearby Attractions

Blue Run Park at the Rainbow River in Dunnellon provides river access for paddlers and some short nature trails; a paved bicycle trail is under construction along the Rainbow River: **marioncountyfl.org.** Captain Mike's Lazy River Cruises depart from the dock at Stumpknocker's Restaurant: **lazyrivercruises.com.**

Directions

From I-75, Exit 341 (Belleview/Dunnellon), drive west on CR 484 for 14.5 miles, crossing FL 200 en route. The trailhead is prominently posted on the left-hand side of FL 200 just past the Dunnellon Regional Airport.

Florida Trail: Santos

SCENERY: ★ ★ ★

TRAIL CONDITION: ★ ★ ★ ★ ★

CHILDREN: ★ ★ ★ ★

DIFFICULTY: ★ ★ ★

SOLITUDE: ★ ★

GPS TRAILHEAD COORDINATES:
N29° 06.335' W82° 05.652'

DISTANCE & CONFIGURATION:
3.4-mile out-and-back

HIKING TIME: 1.5 hours

HIGHLIGHTS: Karst features, giant grapevines

ACCESS: Daily, sunrise–sunset; open for backpacking 24/7. Free.

MAPS: USGS *Belleview*, maps at trailhead kiosk

FACILITIES: Restrooms and water fountain at trailhead, adjacent campground

WHEELCHAIR ACCESS: None

COMMENTS: Leashed dogs welcome. Backpackers may use designated campsites with a free permit; call the Sharpes Ferry Office. No permit required for Florida Trail Association members.

CONTACTS: Office of Greenways and Trails, Sharpes Ferry Office: 352-236-7143; **floridahikes.com/florida-trail-cross-florida-greenway.** Florida Trail Association: 352-378-8823; **floridatrail.org**

Overview

The first section of the Florida Trail to open along the Cross Florida Greenway, and by far the busiest trailhead due to its location right off US 441, the Santos section of the Florida Trail on the Cross Florida Greenway adjoins the Santos Campground and the Santos Mountain Biking Trails. This 3.5-mile round-trip to the next road crossing (SE 25th Avenue) is always busy with joggers, runners, and folks walking their dogs or taking their children on short strolls. Since this trail was first established, the surrounding forests have peaked and declined. So you won't see a lot of habitat diversity here. But the rugged karst landscape underfoot makes for some interesting terrain.

Route Details

From the parking area adjoining the restrooms, check the kiosk for a trail map. Walk up to the left side of the restrooms and follow

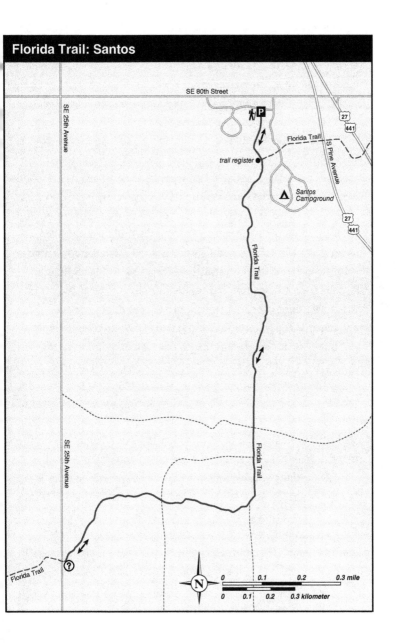

Florida Trail: Santos

SE 80th Street

SE 25th Avenue

Florida Trail

SE Pine Avenue

27
441

trail register

Santos
Campground

27
441

Florida Trail

Florida Trail

SE 25th Avenue

Florida Trail

N

| 0 | 0.1 | 0.2 | 0.3 mile |
| 0 | 0.1 | 0.2 | 0.3 kilometer |

the blue blazes beneath the slash pines through a dense, vine-filled understory. You can see tents and campers in the Santos Campground to the left, and a kiosk and parking for the mountain bikers uphill to the right. The trail heads downhill to meet the orange-blazed Florida Trail. Turn right and you'll find a trail register. Sign in before you start following the orange blazes.

One of the fascinating things about this part of the trail is what is underfoot—rocks. This region is known for its eroded limestone bedrock, called karst. When we were kids, an attraction called Ocala Caverns offered tours nearby. As you turn away from the campground, the trail climbs steadily, with roots and rocks underfoot. You can see parallel trails to right as the Florida Trail meanders beneath hanging mosses and dangling grapevines. The high canopy above is mainly laurel oaks, tall and straight, with a smattering of pines.

There is an elevation change here because of the karst. The trail curves past some cabbage palms, which need water to survive—their roots tap into the water below. Water flows freely beneath the surface here but does not emerge, as this trail is high and dry. In retrospect, it's a very good thing that the Cross Florida Barge Canal never came to fruition, as it would have destroyed the natural flow of freshwater through the Floridan Aquifer, affecting drinking water throughout the region. On the right, the landscape drops off into a deep bowl filled with live oaks. The trail stays atop the limestone bluffs on the rim of the sinkhole while the bike trails drop down into it.

At 0.5 mile you see a path to the right and the sign for PINE TREE TRAIL, part of the mountain biking trails. The Florida Trail swings left, entering a bright and sunny meadow with loblolly pines above and coral bean and blackberries below. The laurel oak forest closes in again. There are many fallen trees and limbs covered in lichens and mosses. Vivid mushrooms, such as the metallic-purple violet cort, thrive in the leaf litter and decaying wood. Laden with resurrection fern, oak branches arch overhead.

As the trail approaches a pine plantation, grapevines thicker than your arms and almost big enough to swing on dangle from the live oaks just within reach, forming loops and swirls above the footpath. The path follows a windbreak of oaks with fenceposts between them, marking the boundary between two farms. Crossing a firebreak, you see a former pasture planted in longleaf pines. Just beyond a mountain bike trail intersection, an enormous oak has fallen across the footpath, and the trail keeper simply cut a path through the log.

At 1.1 miles you cross the equestrian wagon trail, here a sand road, at marker E-10. The understory is extremely thick with pokeberry and beautyberry. After a dip in the footpath, it continues along the line of oaks. Warblers add layers of melody to the forest canopy. It's surprising, despite how close this trail starts to US 441, that the forest absorbs enough road noise to provide a pocket of solitude at this point.

Despite the quiet, you're not alone. With a series of trail intersections coming up, starting with the wagon trail again at marker E-12, you're apt to see equestrians and cyclists coming and going in several directions, especially on the weekends. Pine needles carpet the footpath for a brief stretch as it leads you over an undulating forest floor, perhaps once a planted field. Where you see a small clearing beneath a stand of pines, there is a gopher tortoise burrow nearby. Fall wildflowers paint this corner of the understory in hues of purple and yellow.

The trails begin to converge, and you see a paved road to the right. This is SE 25th Avenue, the turnaround point for this hike. A kiosk is on this side of the road, along with a bench. On the other side of the road is trailhead parking used for the Vortex Trails, a series of mountain biking loops that dip into a deep quarry with a cave in the bottom.

After 1.7 miles you've reached the end of the Santos section, although the Florida Trail continues west for another 4.9 miles to the Land Bridge Trailhead. Turn around and return along the same footpath, following the orange blazes. Pay special attention on the return trip to the trail crossings so as not to wander off on one of the mountain biking trails.

By 3 miles you're walking uphill from the limestone bluff along the sinkhole. You start to hear road noise and encounter rocks and roots underfoot. When you see the fence on the right along the campground, you know your walk is almost complete. At the trail junction with its trail register and directional sign, turn left to follow the blue blazes back to the parking area. Returning to the kiosk at the parking area, you've completed a 3.4-mile hike.

Nearby Attractions

The award-winning Santos Mountain Biking Trails are full of surprises as they dip deeper into the karst features you sampled along the hike: **omba.org.** Rentals are available nearby at Greenway Bicycles (**greenwaybicycles.blogspot.com**) and Santos Bike Shop (**santosbikeshop.com**). Learn to cave dive in a karst window—a peek into the Floridan Aquifer—at Paradise Springs, southeast on US 441: **geocities.ws/paradisespringsfla.**

Directions

From I-75, Exit 341 (Belleview/Dunnellon), drive east on FL 484 to the first traffic light. Turn left on CR 475A, and drive 2.8 miles north, passing the Land Bridge Trailhead (Hike 29). At the next right turn, CR 475B, turn right and continue 1.1 mile east to the T intersection with CR 475. Turn left and drive north 2.8 miles to SE 80th Street. Turn right and continue east 2.5 miles to the second Santos Trailhead entrance (the first is for the mountain biking trails) on the right. The intersection of SE 80th Street and US 441 is just past the trailhead entrance at the traffic light. It is located 3 miles north of downtown Belleview and 6.4 miles south of downtown Ocala, with the Santos Sheriff Station a prominent landmark.

28

Florida Trail:

Southwest 49th Avenue to Land Bridge

SCENERY: ★ ★ ★ ★ ★
TRAIL CONDITION: ★ ★ ★ ★
CHILDREN: ★ ★
DIFFICULTY: ★ ★ ★ ★ ★
SOLITUDE: ★ ★ ★ ★

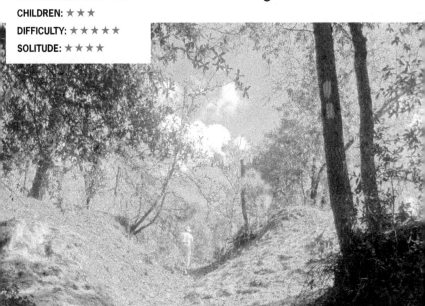

CLAMBERING UP THE OLD DIGGINGS NEAR SW 49TH AVENUE

GPS TRAILHEAD COORDINATES: N29° 02.461' W82° 12.068'

DISTANCE & CONFIGURATION: 5.7-mile balloon

HIKING TIME: 3 hours

HIGHLIGHTS: Rugged terrain, Cross Florida Barge Canal diggings

ACCESS: Daily, sunrise–sunset; open for backpacking 24/7. Free.

MAPS: USGS *Shady,* on kiosk

FACILITIES: Portable toilet and picnic area at trailhead; benches, kiosks, and campsite along the trail

WHEELCHAIR ACCESS: None

COMMENTS: Leashed dogs welcome. Backpackers may use designated campsites with a free permit; call the Sharpes Ferry Office. No permit required for Florida Trail Association members.

CONTACTS: Office of Greenways and Trails, Sharpes Ferry Office: 352-236-7143; **floridahikes.com/florida-trail-cross-florida-greenway.** Florida Trail Association: 352-378-8823; **floridatrail.org.**

Florida Trail: SW 49th Avenue to Land Bridge

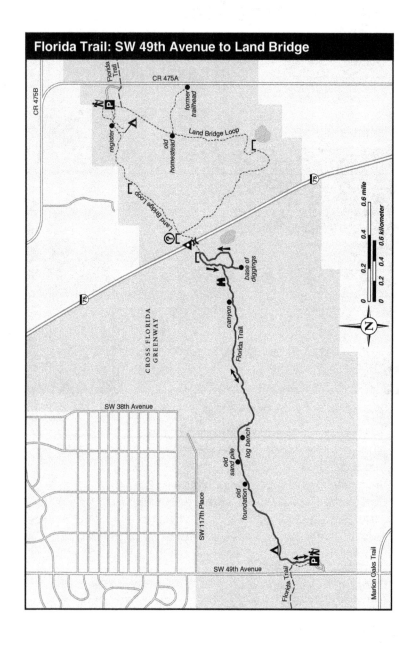

Overview

With nearly 6 miles of rugged hiking along the Cross Florida Greenway, the Florida Trail between the Southwest 49th Avenue Trailhead and the Land Bridge is a lesson in Florida's environmental history and the healing power of time. Native habitats reclaimed one of Florida's largest public works projects, the Cross Florida Barge Canal, with time and erosion creating the steep ravines and bluffs that the trail now traverses. The loop portion of this hike lets you see what remains of this big dig, as well as peek at the renowned Land Bridge over I-75.

Route Details

Starting at the trailhead kiosk, follow the blue blazes. It's a little confusing as you see mountain bike signage right away, so watch for a FT sign beyond the OMBA sign, and follow the FT path into the sandhills, the turkey oak leaves making crunching sounds underfoot as you walk. Crossing a limerock road, the blue-blazed trail leads you into a scrubby habitat with big drops off the footpath. You descend a steep slope with roots sticking out like a staircase. The sides are hard-packed sand, but there are enough pine needles that you can slip and slide.

At a quarter mile you reach the Florida Trail junction. Turn right at the sign to start walking east toward the Land Bridge. A steep ascent follows through a cut. A primitive campsite with a picnic bench is atop the bluff, a short blue-blazed trail leading to it. The main trail stays to the right. Now that you've made your first traverse across the former barge canal—for decades a giant, deep gash in Florida's landscape until the forests filled it in—the trail levels out, easing into the natural undulations of the sandhill habitat.

The trail enters a sand pine forest. The extensive sand pine forest along this trek is why this section of the Cross Florida Greenway has been dubbed "Christmas" on the maps, as the soft-needled young sand pines make nice Christmas trees. Crossing the limerock wagon road, the trail heads downhill. Fallen logs line the footpath through one area. Bracken fern noses out of the leafy duff on the forest floor.

Reaching the limerock road again, the trail slips into a forest of tall, slender sand pines so close together they feel like a wall of bamboo.

At 0.9 mile the trail crosses the corner of a foundation of a small square building surrounded by the forest. The sand pines just beyond grow incredibly large and tall for a species whose normal life span is no more than 60 years. Shield lichens drape from upper limbs. There are fungal galls on limbs and trunks, some large enough to mistake for a hornet's nest. As the trail heads downhill into a scrub forest, you can see a distant ridge topped with pines through a break in the canopy on the left. Just before you meet the limerock road again, a fallen piece of sand pine has been smoothed off as a natural log bench.

Beneath the gnarled branches of sand live oak, the trail ascends and descends, dancing along the rim of the big dig, which drops off sharply to your right. In this scrub forest, notice the many delicate lichens that grow in patches of soft sand. One of the more unusual species here is *Cladonia prostrata.* Dry, it has a nubby popcorn look. Sprinkle a little water on it, and it unfurls to look like a miniature staghorn fern.

As the trail climbs upward again, you enter a stand of taller pines. Passing Florida rosemary, the trail continues its plunges and scrambles through a tight corridor of sand live oaks covered in brilliant lichens and mosses. Atop one ridge, the habitat transitions from scrub into a forest of tall loblolly pines. The trail drops off the ridge to the right into the canal diggings. At 2.1 miles you enter an area reminiscent of the southern Appalachians. This side of the diggings is deeply carved by decades of rain into a series of steep drainages beneath the pines. Watch for the double blazes as they guide you through this maze of clumps of earth covered in forest.

At an obvious fork in the trail, the unmarked fork to the right leads down to a terrace. It overlooks the forest in the bottom of the canal bed. Scramble back up and continue to follow the orange blazes. Depending on the tree cover and time of year, you can see across to the far side of the canal, the earth a yellowish-orange in the distance.

By 2.4 miles you reach a bench. Take the trail to the right of the bench. It is unmarked but well maintained, and is the beginning of the loop down into the diggings. As it drops into the canal basin, you hear interstate traffic in the distance. Passing the back side of a sign, No Horses Beyond This Point, cross the limerock road and follow the equestrian trail marked E-80 to see the historic diggings. There are two benches and a junction of trails at its base. Since the trails were first established in 1999, I've watched the vegetation fill it in, but it still looks like a giant sand dune and is the only place along the Cross Florida Greenway like this. The horse trail continues up and over the "dune" so it's fine to walk up it and let the kids roll down it.

Leaving the diggings, walk back to the limerock road and make a right at the No Horses sign. Follow the road to leave the bottom of the canal. The road curves to the left and ascends into sand pine forest, the sound of traffic increasing. By 2.9 miles you reach the big Land Bridge sign. All of the trails merge here to cross the bridge. Walk out to the center of the bridge to the overlook. It's the same destination you can access from the Land Bridge Loop (Hike 29) but from the opposite side of I-75.

Retrace your steps down the bridge on the west side. As you pass the limestone watering trough, you'll see the FT sign marking the Florida Trail. Turn right to follow the orange blazes. This loop portion of the trail continues through the sand pine scrub, here dense with diminutive oaks in the understory. Prickly pear cactus and Florida rosemary grow in sandy spots along this narrow footpath. Crossing a perpendicular pathway, scramble up into the denser forest, where resurrection fern grows along the trunk of a cedar tree.

Walking through the tightly knit oaks, you reach the bench at 3.3 miles, completing the loop. As you spend the next hour scrambling in and out of the well-eroded north side of this abandoned canal, consider the backbreaking work expended by thousands of unemployed Floridians working for the Works Progress Administration in 1935, digging this ditch with shovels, using mules to cart away and pile up the soil. While the canal—an environmental nightmare—thankfully never came to pass, all of that hard work produced this unusually rugged terrain for hiking. Following the trail back the way you came, be sure to turn off onto the blue-blazed side trail once you descend the steep bluff just past the campsite. You return to the Southwest 49th Avenue Trailhead for a 5.7-mile hike.

Nearby Attractions

At I-75, Exit 341, the Don Garlits Auto Museums showcase antique cars, dragsters, and racing memorabilia from the man who popularized drag racing: **garlits.com.**

Directions

From I-75, Exit 341 (Belleview/Dunnellon), drive west 2.3 miles on CR 484 to the second traffic light. Turn right on Marion Oaks Course at the traffic light. Follow it 0.8 mile as it curves and becomes Marion Oaks Trail. Turn right on SW 49th Avenue and continue 0.4 mile. The trailhead is on the right.

29

Land Bridge Loop

SCENERY: ★ ★ ★ ★
TRAIL CONDITION: ★ ★ ★ ★
CHILDREN: ★ ★ ★ ★
DIFFICULTY: ★ ★
SOLITUDE: ★ ★

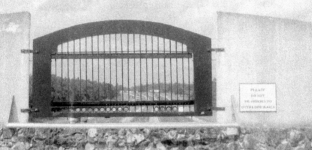

LOOKING DOWN ON INTERSTATE 75 FROM THE LAND BRIDGE

GPS TRAILHEAD COORDINATES: N29° 02.461' W82° 12.068'

DISTANCE & CONFIGURATION: 3.5-mile loop

HIKING TIME: 1.5 hours

HIGHLIGHTS: Ancient oak trees, crossing the Land Bridge over I-75

ACCESS: Daily, sunrise–sunset; open for backpacking 24/7. Free.

MAPS: USGS *Shady*, on trailhead kiosk

FACILITIES: Restrooms and water fountain at trailhead; benches, kiosks, and primitive campsite along the trail loop

WHEELCHAIR ACCESS: None

COMMENTS: Leashed dogs welcome. Backpackers may use designated campsites with a free permit; call the Sharpes Ferry Office. No permit required for Florida Trail Association members.

CONTACTS: Office of Greenways and Trails, Sharpes Ferry Office: 352-236-7143; **floridahikes.com/florida-trail-cross-florida-greenway.** Florida Trail Association: 352-378-8823; **floridatrail.org.**

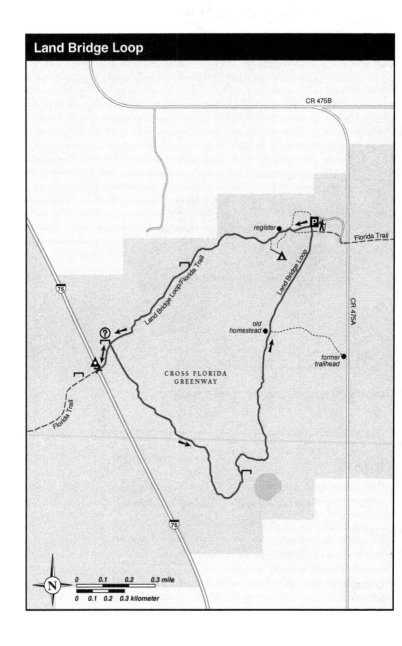

Land Bridge Loop

CR 475B

register

Florida Trail

Land Bridge Loop/Florida Trail

Land Bridge Loop

75

CR 475A

old
homestead

former
trailhead

CROSS FLORIDA
GREENWAY

Florida Trail

75

0   0.1   0.2   0.3 mile

0   0.1 0.2   0.3 kilometer

N

Overview

Since its construction began in 1999, the Land Bridge has been a prominent feature along I-75 south of Ocala. Modeled after similar designs in the Netherlands, it is a giant planter of native vegetation, providing a natural surface for hikers, cyclists, equestrians, and wildlife to cross the interstate along the Cross Florida Greenway. One of the more popular trails in the region, the 3.5-mile Land Bridge Loop—made up of the Florida Trail and a former section of the Florida Trail—provides an easy, mostly shaded walk to see this civil engineering marvel up close.

Route Details

Under the shade of large live oaks, the trail begins at an FT sign at a pass-through in the fence. Following the orange blazes, you immediately pass the blue-blazed trail, the return loop, coming in from the left. This linear forest of live oaks, which includes some very showy trees, provided a windbreak between farmers' fields. After you step through the limbs of an oak that touches the ground, look left to see a split oak with a side trail right through its middle. Crossing the wagon trail used by equestrians, you encounter a trail register. Sign in here.

You'll walk across several intersections with equestrian and mountain biking trails—all of which are also accessed through the Land Bridge Trailhead—before you see a blue-blazed trail to the left. It leads to a primitive campsite with a picnic table, bench, and fire ring. As you walk through the forest of tall laurel oaks, you spy young longleaf pines bathed in sunlight in a restored pasture to the left, and a handful of turkey oaks, which are particularly resplendent in fall. Reaching the corner of a fence line along a horse farm, the trail curves left to go around it. A mountain bike trail draws close on the right. An equestrian trail comes in from the left. Reaching a park bench beneath a canopy of live oaks, you've hiked 0.6 mile.

After a few more trail crossings, the understory of the forest becomes thick with vegetation, particularly grapevines and young oaks. Pine needles begin to carpet the trail, forming a cushy walking surface, and dangle from branches and leaves like tinsel. Giant grape-vines drape from the trees above. Fungi flourish on and around the remains of rotting logs, while puffs of deer moss grow atop the pine needles on the forest floor. Traffic noise picks up as the trail corridor closes in tightly. As you gain a little elevation, you start to see sand pines and myrtle oaks, indicators of scrub habitat—confirmed when you hit patches of soft sand underfoot.

The footpath emerges at the equestrian road at 1.1 miles and turns right, passing a kiosk with a bench and a junction of all the trails, including the blue-blazed return trail. Continue past the kiosk to the LAND BRIDGE sign and follow the limerock road up the bridge for a look at the bridge. Dedicated on National Trails Day in June 2000, this was America's first true land bridge. More than a thousand tons of material went into its construction, a design capable of hold-ing an atypical weight of rocks, soil, water, and growing trees. Over-looks in the center let visitors wave to the traffic below.

After your visit to the Land Bridge, return to the kiosk where all the trails meet. A map is posted here showing the overall route. Your return is along the original Florida Trail route, now blazed in blue. The trail forks immediately; stay to the right, where there is a HIKING ONLY sign. Longleaf pines tower overhead. In fall, you see bright dashes of yellow-orange from hickory trees.

The trail heads south, paralleling the interstate—not visible, but noisy. After crossing Equestrian Trail 2 at 1.6 miles, the under-story closes in with dense young growth. Beyond a gopher tortoise burrow, the trail is edged with saw palmetto. The oaks in the high canopy above are canted in crazy directions as the forest ages and falls. American holly, sweetgum, and silk bay create a lower canopy. You pass an oak with a massive gall on its side. To the left is a clearing with a small pond, barely discernible through the riot of vegetation.

Passing a bench at 2.3 miles, the trail continues through a tan-gle of young oaks. Creating the high canopy, massive live oaks are laden with Spanish moss, their limbs covered in resurrection fern, a furry green after a rain. Look for delicate greenfly orchids hidden in the ferns—but don't spend all your time gazing upward or you'll trip over roots. After another intersection with Equestrian Trail 2, a pile of limestone rocks nudges into the footpath. Crossing more mountain bike trails, you emerge into former pastureland, now a young longleaf pine forest. Along the mowed path are wizened trees with crazy crooked limbs: Chickasaw plums, native fruit trees that burst into beautiful white blooms by February. The understory is full of blackberry brambles trying to reach out and snag your pants. Hike this trail in late spring to sample their juicy berries.

After passing through a shady hammock created by a cluster of sand live oaks, the trail continues down a mowed path up to the next cluster of trees. At 3 miles the blue-blazed trail forks. To the right, it heads to the former trailhead. Walk a short way down it to inspect the remains of an old homestead site. Return to the intersection and continue on the main trail. As you walk the mowed path, you can feel the undulations of the former plow lines underfoot.

Passing under the shade of a cherry tree, the trail crosses a two-track road. Coming up to a Florida Trail marker, you can see the line of live oaks up ahead. Crossing an equestrian trail, follow the blue blazes along the fence line to complete the 3.5-mile loop, and turn right to exit.

Nearby Attractions

Gypsy Gold offers tours at its breeding facility for showy Gypsy Vanner horses: **gypsygold.com.** Off CR 475, the Florida Horse Park is a major competitive training facility that offers on-site camping and trail rides: **flhorsepark.com.**

Directions

From I-75, Exit 341 (Belleview/Dunnellon), drive east on FL 484 to the first traffic light. Turn left on CR 475A and continue 2 miles north. Turn left at the trailhead entrance, following the entrance road as it sweeps past the equestrian parking area to the parking area set farther back near the restrooms.

SCENERY: ★ ★ ★ ★
TRAIL CONDITION: ★ ★ ★
CHILDREN: ★ ★ ★
DIFFICULTY: ★ ★
SOLITUDE: ★ ★ ★

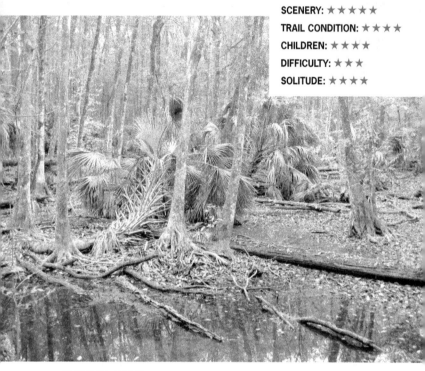

MARSHALL SWAMP

GPS TRAILHEAD COORDINATES: N29° 11.024' W82° 00.966'

DISTANCE & CONFIGURATION: 4.5-mile balloon

HIKING TIME: 2 hours

HIGHLIGHTS: Old-growth trees, junglelike setting, willow pond

ACCESS: Daily, sunrise–sunset. Free.

MAPS: USGS *Ocala East,* maps at kiosk

FACILITIES: Restrooms and water fountain at trailhead; benches along trail loop, picnic bench at turnaround point

WHEELCHAIR ACCESS: None

COMMENTS: Leashed dogs welcome. Use bug spray; mosquitoes can be fierce. Boardwalks may be slippery.

CONTACTS: Office of Greenways and Trails, Sharpes Ferry Office: 352-236-7143; **floridahikes.com/florida-trail-cross-florida-greenway.** Florida Trail Association: 352-378-8823; **floridatrail.org.**

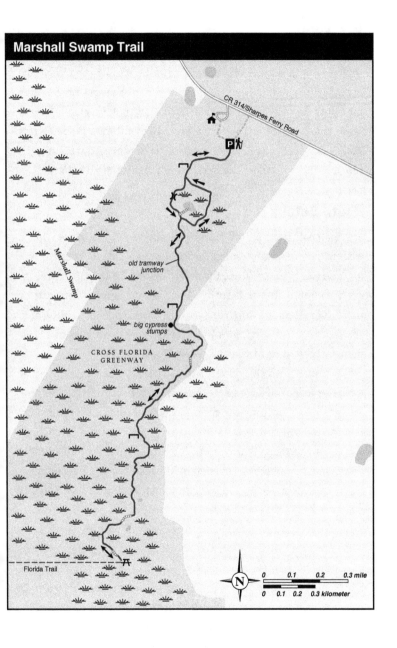

Marshall Swamp Trail

CR 314/Sharpes Ferry Road

Marshall Swamp

old tramway
junction

big cypress
stumps

CROSS FLORIDA
GREENWAY

Florida Trail

N

| 0 | 0.1 | 0.2 | 0.3 mile |

| 0 | 0.1 | 0.2 | 0.3 kilometer |

Overview

Encompassing more than 12,000 acres of floodplain forest, Marshall Swamp is a massive natural landform defining the Ocklawaha River basin upstream from the Silver River. In the part of the swamp protected by the Cross Florida Greenway, the Marshall Swamp Trail—most of which is also a linear portion of the statewide Florida Trail—immerses you in this virtual jungle of oversized trees and the fungi, ferns, and other flora that flourish in this humid habitat.

Route Details

The Marshall Swamp Trail starts adjacent to the trail kiosk, with a well-defined footpath leading through into an upland forest. Crossing a service road, you'll see the first of several TRAIL signs confirming your route. The trail surface is compacted gravel, softened by more than a decade's worth of grasses, mosses, and pine needles atop the footpath. Loblolly pines tower above a lower canopy of sweetgum, hickory, and red maple, a showcase of fall color.

Passing a bench, you reach the LOOP TRAIL sign on the left at a quarter mile. You'll complete the loop on the return trip. Continue straight ahead, noticing the enormous loblolly pine. One of the best reasons to do this hike is to see the truly ancient trees throughout this forest, particularly the pines. Crossing a bridge over the outflow of a cypress swamp, the trail enters Marshall Swamp, the landform named for an antebellum sugar plantation that stood a little north of here along the Ocklawaha River.

A side trail to the left leads to a boardwalk with an observation deck on a small willow pond frequented by large frogs. Returning to main trail, you come to the second Loop Trail junction at a bench at a half mile. Pass this and continue on the main orange-blazed trail. Hear that rustle under the cabbage palms? It's probably an armadillo. As you go deeper into the swamp, keep alert for wildlife. Pileated woodpeckers call to each other in the high canopy.

While the trail is rarely soggy underfoot, you'll see low-lying spots on both sides where water collects in the remains of rotted-out root balls. This is a humid place, where sphagnum moss swarms up the trunks of cabbage palms and pine trees. More large pines tower overhead. Grapevines as thick as a boa constrictor dangle from above. This is truly Tarzan territory—many of the Johnny Weissmuller movies were filmed just a few miles from here.

Passing an old tramway on the left, you're reminded of the human legacy in ancient forests: most of the old-growth cypresses were logged out of this swamp more than half a century ago. Straight ahead is a massive swamp chestnut oak with shaggy bark, huge leaves, and a buttressed trunk to anchor itself deep in the muck. Bromeliads thrive in the high branches of the trees. Beyond a bench at 0.9 mile, notice the thickness of lichens on the tree trunks, as if painted on in multiple coats.

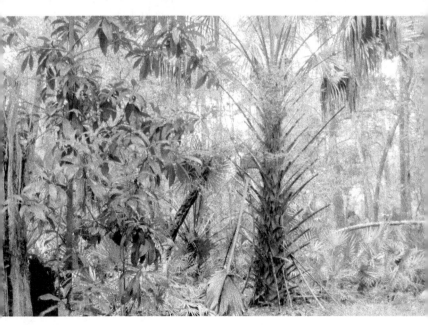

PALMS, MAGNOLIAS, AND TALL HARDWOODS DOMINATE THE FOREST AT MARSHALL SWAMP

When the trail first opened, the tree canopy still blotted out the sky. Since then, a combination of pine bark beetle infestation and the loss of trees during hurricanes has enabled rays of sunlight to reach the forest floor in scattered spots. Unfortunately, near the 1-mile mark, there is a new gash in this ancient forest—a fence erected by a private company that bought part of the swamp and carved a swath down it to mark their territory. I'm told that this trail may move away from the fence at some point, but the swamp is deeper in that direction, so it will take some time. Meanwhile, as you walk, focus your attention away from the fence line and into the dense swamp to your right and its impassive understory, capped with towering cypress trees. At 1.2 miles you reach a boardwalk for the outflow of the cypress swamp, with a bench not long afterward. As cypress knees creep right up to both sides of the trail, you know you're in the swamp. The footpath may flood through this section. The cypresses here are not only tall, but their bases are also heavily buttressed. Look carefully at those scrapes on the cypress bark: you might see the claw marks of a Florida black bear.

Swaddled in mosses and fungi, the root balls of cabbage palms swell in size. Every log is covered in lichens and fungi, with some forming natural planters for ferns. Sweetgums rain down colorful leaves each fall into a sluggish stream, where a boardwalk arches through the cypress swamp past cypress knees so tall they seem out of proportion. A bench after the boardwalk is at the 2-mile mark of the hike. Old cypress stumps—what is left after logging—hide under the giant fronds of young cabbage palms. More tall trees tower overhead.

Thickly carpeted with fallen leaves, the final boardwalk leads you into a small upland area. At 2.2 miles you reach the picnic table, which marks the end of the Marshall Swamp Trail at a T intersection with a tramway. The Florida Trail continues down the tramway to the right on its way to the Baseline Road Trailhead, but this is your turnaround point, a good stop for hydration and a snack.

Retracing your walk through Marshall Swamp, pay attention to the sounds of the forest: a symphony of songbirds, the clatter of woodpeckers, the rustle of palm fronds in the breeze. After 3.9 miles you return to the Loop Trail junction. Turn right to follow the blue-blazed Loop Trail through the upland forest around the willow pond. At the T intersection with a tramway, turn left to follow the trail past the LOOP TRAIL sign. The trail goes over a culvert draining the pond into the swamp.

As the trail rises up into pine forest, keep alert for deer. Behind the sabal palm marker on the right is the largest loblolly pine you'll see on this hike, and it's certainly impressive. You reach the old LOOP TRAIL sign, and it points you left past the new sign, down a narrow corridor crowded on both sides by grapevines and saw palmetto. Reaching a T intersection with the back side of the first LOOP TRAIL sign, you've completed the loop. Turn right to exit, finishing your hike at the trail kiosk after 4.5 miles.

Nearby Attractions

Just up the road, Silver Springs State Park (Hikes 37 and 38) offers hiking trails, camping, and paddling on the Silver River, plus access to Silver Springs and its world-famous glass-bottomed boats: **floridastateparks.org/silversprings.** With newly established hiking trails, Indian Lake State Forest is north of Silver Springs along CR 35: **floridaforestservice.com.**

Directions

From I-75, Exit 352 (Ocala), take FL 40 for 8.4 miles east through downtown Ocala to Silver Springs. Turn south on CR 35/Baseline Road, and drive 1.5 miles to the traffic light at CR 314/Sharpes Ferry Road. Turn left and continue 2 miles to the trailhead entrance on the right, just past the Office of Greenways and Trails, Sharpes Ferry Office.

Ocala and Vicinity (Hikes 31–38)

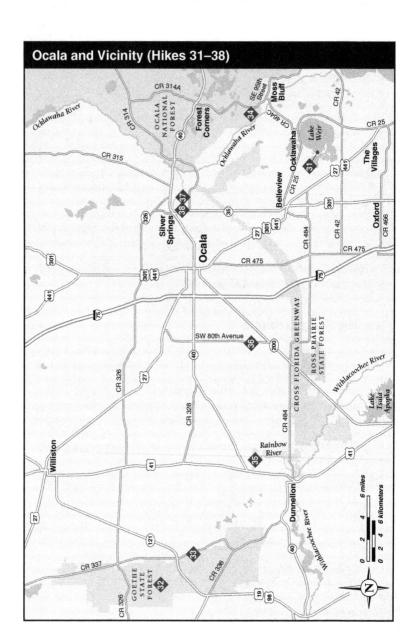

Ocala & Vicinity

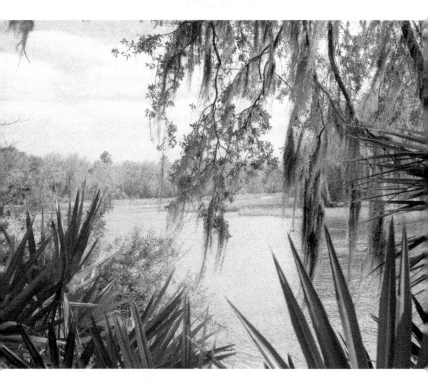

RAINBOW RIVER; *see Hike 35, page 231*

Carney Island Recreation & Conservation Area

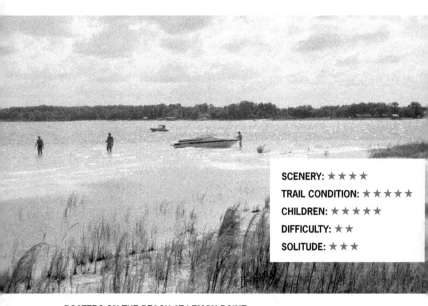

SCENERY: ★ ★ ★ ★
TRAIL CONDITION: ★ ★ ★ ★ ★
CHILDREN: ★ ★ ★ ★ ★
DIFFICULTY: ★ ★
SOLITUDE: ★ ★ ★

BOATERS ON THE BEACH AT LEMON POINT

GPS TRAILHEAD COORDINATES: N29° 00.890' W81° 57.876'

DISTANCE & CONFIGURATION: 3.8-mile balloon

HIKING TIME: 1.5 hours

HIGHLIGHTS: Ancient live oaks, beach at Lemon Point

ACCESS: Daily, sunrise–sunset. Entrance fee: $5 per vehicle.

MAPS: USGS *Lake Weir*, at trailhead kiosk

FACILITIES: Restrooms and water fountain, playground, and picnic area at trailhead; swimming beach nearby. Benches and covered platforms along the trail loop.

WHEELCHAIR ACCESS: None

COMMENTS: Pets not permitted. Bicycles not permitted. Wildlife sightings are best in the early morning, before other visitors arrive. Beware of fire ant nests on the edges of the trail.

CONTACTS: Carney Island Recreation & Conservation Area: 352-671-8560; **marioncounty fl.org/Parks/Pr_Directory/Park_Carney.aspx**. Marion County Parks and Recreation: **marion countyfl.org**.

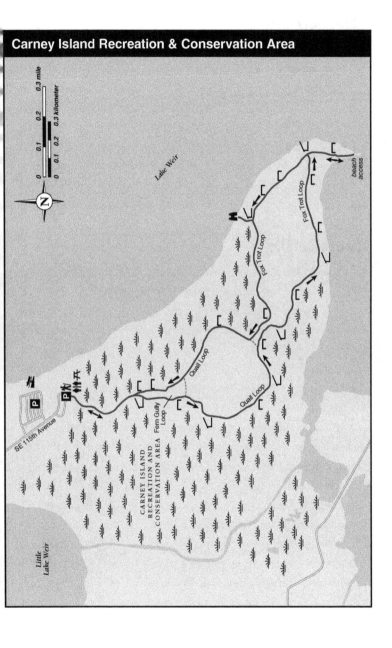

Overview

The breeze carries the scent of orange blossoms from some of the northernmost remaining commercial groves in Florida. Lake Weir is a palatable presence, more than 5,800 acres of wet shallows favored by anglers and paddlers. Covered with citrus groves from 1875 through the 1990s, Carney Island is a peninsula jutting out into the lake, the conservation area covering 750 acres of old-growth live oak hammocks, floodplain forests, sandhills, and agricultural lands under restoration. The trail system lets you imagine what it felt like to walk a country road a century ago in this part of Florida.

Route Details

Walk up to the kiosk just beyond the edge of the parking area. It's the junction of two trails, a connector to the swimming area on Little Lake Weir and the main trail system, which is made up of three stacked loops. This hike follows the perimeter of the loops, beginning with the Fern Gully Trail. Leaving the beautiful oak hammock that surrounds the picnic area, it follows a causeway into a floodplain forest that drains into Lake Weir. The width of the trail is that of a road, and you'll see tire tracks in it from the park rangers and from the occasional special event when a tram runs around the loop. However, the feel is that of walking back in time, to the heyday of Florida's orange groves. As you come to the junction for the loop, keep right, passing a covered bench. Ferns flourish in the damp soil between the live oaks. Wild citrus grows throughout the woods, filling the air with perfume each winter. Songbirds flit through the trees.

As the trail curves, it's grassy and open under the oak trees. Coming around the curve, you see a park bench with an interpretive sign next to it and the next trail junction at 0.5 mile. The Fern Gully Trail makes a return loop to the left. Continue straight ahead to start along the Quail Loop. Here, the forest between the trails has been logged, so it's somewhat messy, filled with tall grasses, a few oaks, and cabbage palms. On the right is an enormous live oak lying on its side but still alive. You can walk up to it and take a look.

Ascending a rise, the trail returns to the shade of the live oaks, passing another covered shelter. Watch for wildlife through this section. We've seen fox squirrels, deer, and a flock of wild turkey stroll past. You pass a former gate in a fence and can see the winding of the path ahead. Beyond the next bench, there is another shelter with a SUDDEN DROPOFF sign behind it, a pit filled with vegetation. Stepping into the shade of a spectacular stand of ancient live oaks, you reach the return loop for the Quail Loop at 1 mile. Continue straight ahead to begin the Fox Trot Loop. The tracks of lizards and turkeys stand out in the soft, white sand.

Beyond the next shelter is a pine plantation, slash pines growing in rows with a dense understory beneath them. Along a curve in the trail, a bench provides shade. You start to see a ribbon of blue on the right: Lake Weir. Curving past an interpretive marker on Southern magnolia, the trail reaches the next shelter by 1.4 miles. Walking with views of the lake and the tip of this peninsula, Lemon Point, you enjoy the perpetual breeze across the water. Once the floodplain forest shields the lake from view, watch for the next shelter area. Behind it is a narrow trail, a real footpath, leading to the end of the peninsula. Edged by poison ivy in spots, the trail follows a narrow causeway in the forest. Passing a bench, you work your way between the grapevines and trees, popping out onto the beach at Lemon Point at 2 miles. It's a beauty spot, often occupied on weekends by boaters relaxing on the shore. A shallow marsh edges one side of the peninsula; the water of Lake Weir is clear and inviting.

Return the way you came to get back to the Fox Trot Loop at the shelter and continue along the loop. As the sand gets softer underfoot, it's tough to keep traction as you ascend a slight rise. Walk in the mowed grass beside the trail if the footing is rough. As you pass the next bench, it's obvious the trail is on a bluff above the lake, with glimpses of blue through a screen of forest. A shelter on the right has a path behind it leading down to the marshy edge of the lake, a place to take a peek. Scramble back up and return to the main trail.

Passing some tall, skinny cabbage palms, the trail comes to another shaded bench under a canopy of oaks. By 2.9 miles you've completed the Fox Trot Loop and rejoin the other side of the Quail Loop, with an immersion in the more beautiful side of the ancient live oak hammock. The trail curves away from the oaks and back past the forest under restoration in the middle of the loop. By 3.4 miles you reach the end of the Quail Loop, and you're back on the Fern Gully Trail again. A large sign says RETURN TO TRAILHEAD to point the way.

Passing this cluster of large live oaks, the trail continues with dense forest on both sides. Spanish moss drapes from the oaks shading the footpath. You pass a bench next to an interpretive sign on eastern coral snakes. At the next shelter, you've reached the end of the final loop. Continue straight down the causeway through the floodplain forest to return to the kiosk at the trailhead, finishing your hike after 3.8 miles.

Nearby Attractions

Infamous as the location of the shootout between the FBI and Ma Barker in 1935, Ocklawaha has a fish camp old enough to have served the gangsters, Gator Joe's, established in 1926: **gatorjoesocala.com.** Lake Weir is known for its sandy beaches, not just at Carney Island but also at Johnson Beach (at Gator Joe's) and Hampton Beach: **marion countyfl.org/Parks/Pr_Directory/Park_Hampton.aspx.**

Directions

From I-75, Exit 341, follow CR 484 east 8.2 miles to Belleview. Continue across US 27/301/441, and the road becomes FL 25. Drive another 5.5 miles east to SE 115th Avenue, where you will see a CARNEY ISLAND PARK sign. Turn right. Continue 2.1 miles down this road, which enters the park at the admission gate and ends at the parking area farthest out along the peninsula.

32 Goethe State Forest:
Big Cypress Trail

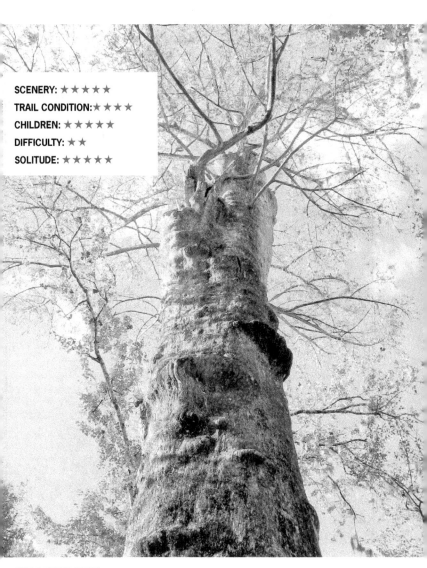

SCENERY: ★ ★ ★ ★ ★
TRAIL CONDITION: ★ ★ ★ ★
CHILDREN: ★ ★ ★ ★ ★
DIFFICULTY: ★ ★
SOLITUDE: ★ ★ ★ ★ ★

THE GOETHE GIANT

Goethe State Forest: Big Cypress Trail

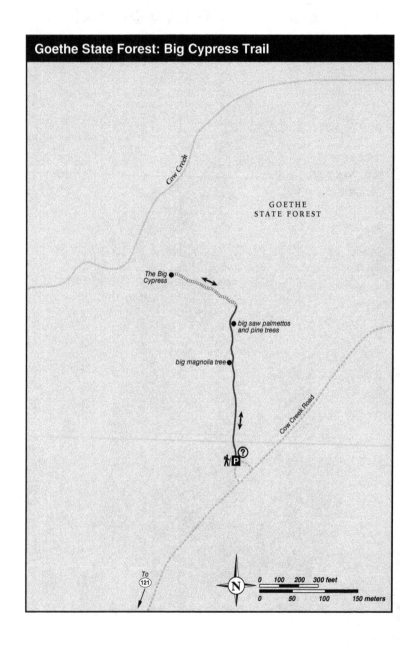

GPS TRAILHEAD COORDINATES: N29° 13.413' W82° 37.360'

DISTANCE & CONFIGURATION: 0.6-mile out-and-back

HIKING TIME: 20 minutes

HIGHLIGHTS: Ancient trees, including the Goethe Giant; excellent interpretive information

ACCESS: Daily, sunrise–sunset. Free.

MAPS: USGS *Tidewater,* at trailhead kiosk

FACILITIES: Picnic bench at trailhead

WHEELCHAIR ACCESS: None

COMMENTS: Pets welcome. Accessed via unpaved, sometimes rough dirt roads. Mosquitoes can be fierce, depending on time of day and time of year.

CONTACTS: Goethe State Forest: 352-465-8585; **floridaforestservice.com**

Overview

Hidden deep in Cow Creek Swamp in the heart of Goethe State Forest—a 53,587-acre forest protecting some of Florida's oldest pine trees—the Big Cypress Trail is a short hike with a big payoff. Leading you past trees of increasing height and girth, it ends as a boardwalk to the base of the Goethe Giant, a towering cypress tree more than 900 years old, with other cypresses of similar stature nearby.

Route Details

Starting at the BIG CYPRESS TRAIL sign, this interpretive trail heads downhill toward Cow Creek Swamp. Loblolly pines tower above. Watch out for roots underfoot as you drop down into the transitional zone between pine flatwoods and floodplain swamp. The interpretive markers along the trail call your attention to the variety of trees that grow in this zone between habitats. Many of these trees are quite large, especially the pines. Once belonging to a local logging company, Goethe State Forest was purchased by the State of Florida after the owner, J. T. Goethe, died. Mr. Goethe's holdings included many patches of old-growth forest, and this is one of them.

The trail turns right where an old path goes left into the floodplain, reaching a corridor outlined with saw palmetto as you come up to the interpretive marker for an American hornbeam. One large tree has toppled nearby, leaving a gaping hole in the canopy and a massive root ball to your right. A Southern magnolia overhead, unusually large and magnificent, hosts scores of bromeliads in its branches. Beyond the magnolia, the footpath gets very rooty and rough, and the forest closes in as if you're entering a jungle. You pass a tall loblolly pine with a lightning strike down its side. The saw palmettoes adjoining it grow straight up like cabbage palms. The trail turns to start the boardwalk.

Created with lumber salvaged from trees killed by pine bark beetles, the boardwalk dates back to 2002. You pass an enormous live oak as you start the walk into the swamp, big trees of many species all around you, amazing in their size and girth. Straight ahead is the Goethe Giant, dominating the forest. It's a heck of a tree. From this perspective, before you reach its base, you can see how tall it is. Fallen trees throughout the forest, covered in fungi, are enormous as well.

At the end of the boardwalk, you stand beneath Florida's seventh-largest cypress tree. By its thick girth and squat crown, you can tell the top was sheared off by a hurricane decades or centuries ago. How did it survive the wholesale logging of cypress forests on this coast? Look up. It has several flaws that spared it from the saw-mill, including a deep hole in the trunk a good 50 feet up, where bees buzz. In 2005, the tree, an estimated 907 years old, measured 28.5 feet in circumference and 87.5 feet tall.

At the base of the cypress are stairs leading into the muck of the swamp. If you're prepared for swamp walking—and have the skills to find your way back to this point—there are more large trees to be seen in Cow Creek Swamp. Several large cypresses are visible from this point. However, the swamp is very muddy and sticky and may have deep mud holes, so only the experienced should venture into it.

Turn around and wander back along the same route. Notice how furry the limbs of the live oaks are, heavily laden with resurrec-tion fern and bromeliads. A tall rusty lyonia adjoins the massive mag-nolia tree. Even the grapevines are big. As you walk back up the trail, the wall of swamp is off to the right; in winter, you can see through the canopy to more large cypresses back there. You return to the trail-head after 0.6 mile.

Nearby Attractions

Goethe State Forest offers several long, multiuse trails accessible from CR 337, including Tidewater, Apex, and Black Prong: **florida forestservice.com.** Hike 33, Buck Island Pond Trail, is to the south. You're less than an hour from Cedar Key, a remote Gulf Coast community that's a step back in time and a fine destination for fresh seafood: **cedarkey.org.**

Directions

The trailhead is off FL 121 in Levy County, between Inglis and Williston, northwest of Dunnellon. From Dunnellon, follow CR 40 west to CR 336. Turn right and drive 10.5 miles to the junction with US 19 and FL 121. Turn right on FL 121. Continue 1.2 miles to the unmarked Cow Creek Road on the right. Cow Creek Road is a dirt forest road passable by passenger vehicles but also used by logging trucks. Following it north, stay right at the first fork in the road. Drive 3.2 miles to the well-marked parking area on the left.

33 # Goethe State Forest:
Buck Island Pond Trail

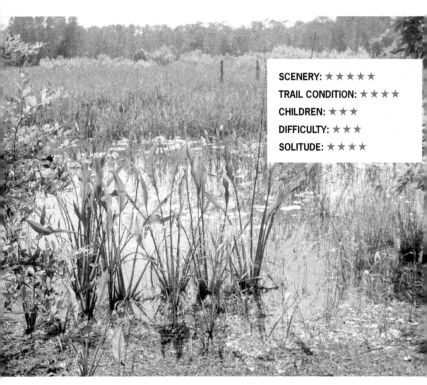

SCENERY: ★ ★ ★ ★
TRAIL CONDITION: ★ ★ ★ ★
CHILDREN: ★ ★
DIFFICULTY: ★ ★
SOLITUDE: ★ ★ ★ ★

BUCK ISLAND POND

GPS TRAILHEAD COORDINATES: N29° 11.003' W82° 34.461'

DISTANCE & CONFIGURATION: 2-mile loop

HIKING TIME: 1.25 hours

HIGHLIGHTS: Observation deck, old-growth pines, pitcher plant bog

ACCESS: Daily, sunrise–sunset. Entrance fee: $2 per person.

MAPS: USGS *Tidewater*, at trailhead kiosk

FACILITIES: Two picnic benches along the loop

WHEELCHAIR ACCESS: None

COMMENTS: Pets welcome. Accessed via unpaved entrance road.

CONTACTS: Goethe State Forest: 352-465-8585; **floridaforestservice.com**

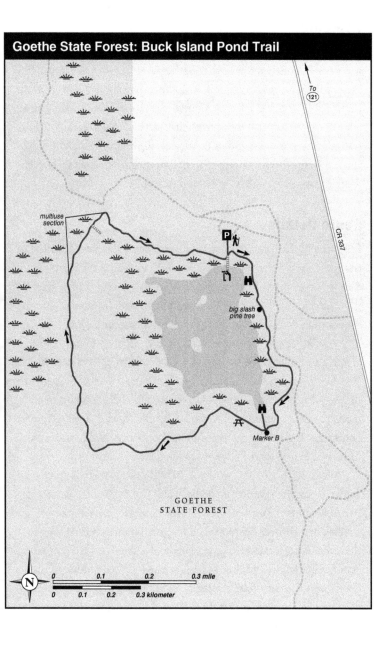

Goethe State Forest: Buck Island Pond Trail

Overview

Looping around a cypress-lined pond in the midst of pine flatwoods, the Buck Island Pond Trail at Goethe State Forest has quite a few interesting features going for it, including a boardwalk to an observation deck that makes it easy for birders to simply sit along the pond's edge and scan avian activity to their heart's content. A walk on the trail may be rewarded with a red-cockaded woodpecker sighting. As the trails are off the beaten path, wildlife encounters are highly probable. Interpretive markers are keyed to a trail map.

Route Details

From the trail kiosk at the parking area, follow the path downhill to the boardwalk. The boardwalk leads to the edge of Buck Island Pond, a large, wet prairie with stretches of open water. Ringed with cypress, the pond attracts many birds, including sandhill cranes. On the observation deck, a picnic table provides a place for birding.

Walk back up the boardwalk and turn right to follow the lime-green blazes clockwise around Buck Island Pond. You pass a NO HORSES sign. Since the trail isn't well known, it's not a beaten path through this section, so you have to watch for blazes. Passing an enormous pine, the trail drops into an oak hammock with scattered pines, descending toward the cypresses along the pond. At the T intersection, turn right to walk to the edge of the pond for another scenic view.

Heading back uphill, you walk beneath the gnarled limbs of sand live oaks, passing a twin-trunked slash pine. Farther uphill, pine plantation surrounds the entrance road. Pines dominate the habitat—fallen needles draped over every branch and shrub, pinecones throughout the understory, mounds of pine straw, and a massive slash pine rising over it all. Just beyond it is a sign: BEWARE THE CYPRESS KNEES. Look down. The knees are the tiniest of nubs. But they are in the footpath, and you could trip over them if you don't watch your footing.

Turning right, the trail closely follows the edge of the pond's floodplain, shaded by dahoon holly, oak, and loblolly bay. Rough underfoot, the footpath can flood. Netted chain and cinnamon fern rise from the damp forest floor. Passing an oak tree with goldfoot fern and resurrection fern growing in its crook, the trail goes uphill briefly, headed toward planted pines. Passing within sight of the sand road at a half mile, it drops back down toward the cypresses, reaching the other side of the BEWARE OF CYPRESS KNEES zone. You reach marker B. A spur trail leads downhill to the edge of the pond, where you can see a wood duck box nearby and the sweep of the wetland beyond. One gnarled-looking cypress appears to be quite old.

Return to the main trail and turn right, walking past younger longleaf pines. Just past a picnic table is marker C, for Slash Pine Plantation. You pass a tall clump of saw palmetto as the trail gets farther from the pond. Deer moss forms seafoam-colored clumps on the forest floor. This is a restoration area, where nature takes its course, filling in vegetation blanks for the planted pines that have been removed.

Marker D is for the gopher tortoise, although no burrow is obvious nearby. Sand live oaks and shiny lyonia hint at scrub habitat as the trail gets farther from the pond; the footpath becomes more distinct. At a mile, the trail takes a sharp turn, entering a well-established pine flatwood. A thick understory of saw palmetto edges the footpath, stretching into the distance in both directions. Marker E shows off older saw palmettos. Past an old road headed toward a cypress dome, you see marker F, which points out the red-cockaded woodpecker and its need for mature longleaf pine. Keep alert for these uncommon birds; we spotted one in this section. Near marker G, about the turpentine industry, watch for catfaced pines; they were carved into for the tapping of their sap. The forest floor hosts reindeer moss and shiny blueberry beneath myrtle oak and rusty lyonia.

After 1.5 miles the trail descends toward the Buck Pond floodplain. You see cypresses up ahead as you come to the back side of a sign: HIKERS TO THE LEFT, HORSES TO THE RIGHT, marking the junction of a shared trail. Continue straight ahead as the trail, now multiuse, widens for a bit to get everyone through the bayhead swamp without getting wet. A cypress dome is to the left, with Buck Pond hidden to the right. Marsh ferns grow in the dark, rich earth.

A side trail at marker H leads to a seepage bog with a handful of hooded pitcher plants. These carnivorous plants love the acidity of the pine needles and the constant dampness of the wet flatwoods. Returning to the main trail, turn right, walking through the wet flatwoods. The multiuse trail diverges at a sign. Turn right to stay on the hiking trail. Vegetation crowds in closely, and the footpath is springy from all the pine needles. Be cautious of a false trail junction where the main trail turns left and slips into the saw palmetto. You see a tangle of loblolly bay and cypress on the right. As you come face-to-face with a tall pine, turn right. The footpath transitions to sand underfoot, and you see the boardwalk up ahead. The trail turns left to parallel it. Exit toward the kiosk and parking area, finishing this 2-mile hike.

Nearby Attractions

Goethe State Forest offers several long, multiuse trails accessible from CR 337, including Tidewater, Apex, and Black Prong: **florida forestservice.com.** Hike 32, Big Cypress Trail, is to the north. At the confluence of the Withlacoochee and Rainbow Rivers, Dunnellon has numerous antiques shops in its historic district: **dunnellon.org.**

Directions

The trailhead is off CR 337 in Levy County, between Inglis and Bronson and to the west of Dunnellon. From US 19 between Inglis and Gulf Hammock, take FL 121 north, and turn right on CR 337. Continue south 2.1 miles from that intersection to the trailhead on the right, not far past the park office and the Apex Trailhead. From Dunnellon, follow CR 40 west to CR 336. Turn right and drive 4.1 miles along CR 336. Turn right on CR 337, passing the Tidewater Trailhead soon after the turn. Watch for the BUCK ISLAND POND sign on the left after 4.7 miles. On the dirt road leading to the trailhead parking area, take the right at the T intersection to continue to the parking area.

Ocklawaha Prairie Restoration Area

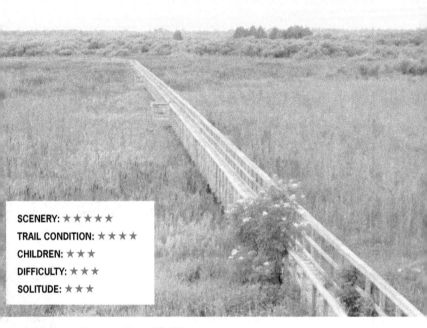

SCENERY: ★ ★ ★ ★ ★

TRAIL CONDITION: ★ ★ ★

CHILDREN: ★ ★

DIFFICULTY: ★ ★ ★

SOLITUDE: ★ ★ ★

BOARDWALK INTO OCKLAWAHA PRAIRIE

GPS TRAILHEAD COORDINATES: N29° 06.357' W81° 54.374'

DISTANCE & CONFIGURATION: 2.5-mile out-and-back

HIKING TIME: 1.25 hours

HIGHLIGHTS: Boardwalk through extensive marshes

ACCESS: Daily, sunrise–sunset. Free.

MAPS: USGS *Lake Weir*, at trailhead kiosk

FACILITIES: Covered pavilion with view, benches along boardwalk

WHEELCHAIR ACCESS: None

COMMENTS: Leashed pets welcome but not advisable on boardwalk portion of the hike. Trailhead is accessed via unpaved roads. Small game and waterfowl hunting is permitted at various times during the year. Check the Florida Fish and Wildlife Conservation Commission website for details: **myfwc.com.**

CONTACTS: St. Johns Water Management District: 386-329-4404; **sjrwmd.com**

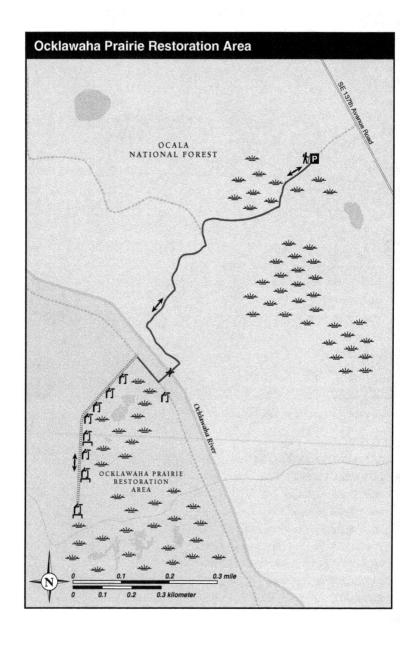

Ocklawaha Prairie Restoration Area

Overview

Flowing north from Lake Griffin, the Ocklawaha River once meandered through vast marshes, cypress swamps, and floodplain forests as it worked its way toward the St. Johns River near Palatka. But channelization by the Army Corps of Engineers radically altered its flow in many places, including around Moss Bluff. At Ocklawaha Prairie Restoration Area, a 6,200-acre preserve east of Lake Weir, restoration of the river floodplain means some of the best wildlife-watching in the region from the edge of a levee and a lengthy boardwalk through the marshes.

Route Details

Your hike starts at the parking area, where you'll find a trail kiosk near a massive Southern magnolia tree. This hike is one of many routes possible through the restoration area but takes you to the heart of its beauty in the Ocklawaha River floodplain. White diamond-shaped markers, typically used to mark horse trails, lead the way.

Walking through the first stand of forest, you can see young longleaf pines up ahead, planted in a former pasture. They're tall enough to generate a little shade. As the trail reaches a T intersection with a grassy strip, turn right. The landscape sweeps to the right down into marshy depressions of floodplain forest. Around 1916, Congress approved draining, diking, and diverting this stretch of the Ocklawaha River into a canal to open up the expansive wetlands to farming and ranching. A dam and levee followed in 1925 at Moss Bluff. Starting in 1973, St. Johns Water Management District began acquiring these farmlands—here and at Sunnyhill Restoration Area, to the south—to restore the wetlands that had been lost along the Ocklawaha River basin.

The main trail junction is at 0.3 mile. To the right, you can see white blazes lead to trails used mainly by equestrians. Turn left, following the sweep of this forest down along the pines. A short distance after you see a sign on the right with a diamond symbol, look to the right and you'll see another one down at the treeline. Follow the grassy path down the hill. Stepping through a narrow swath of floodplain forest on a causeway, you pop out in a patch of old pastureland with young cabbage palms. The trail curves left, entering a stand of sweetgum trees. After the footpath emerges in a sandy area, follow the sweep of sand to the right, where you see the next marker. Clumps of deer moss and masses of reindeer lichen favor this tiny patch of scrub habitat. The trail curves left into a stand of trees, becoming a mowed path. To your right you can see a levee beyond the trees, between you and the open space beyond; it's the C-212 Canal, a deep ditch. Look up, and you'll see a saw palmetto perfectly perched in an unexpected spot, the crook of a live oak tree.

By 0.7 mile the trail ascends a small bluff and meets a road at a T intersection. To the left is private property, The Refuge at Ocklawaha. Turn right and cross the canal on the bridge. The panorama of wetlands in front of you is the Ocklawaha Prairie, the river's historic floodplain. These are vast marshes where thousands of migratory birds spend their winters. Trail maps show that the levee makes a 10.8-mile loop around the prairie, best explored by bike. The destination for this hike, however, is the boardwalk, which you can see out in the marsh.

Turn right and walk down to the boardwalk. You start off down a long straightaway, where obvious indentations in the mat of plants around you mark alligator trails. Depending on the time of year, you'll see different water levels, which favor a different array of plants. In open water, water spangles and water lettuce float on the surface. Late summer brings the brilliant yellows of swamp sunflower. In fall, sea myrtle blooms in cloudlike puffs, and, swaying on their vines, the purple blossoms of climbing aster dance in the breeze. To the west, Carolina willows crowd your view; cypress trees rise from the edge of the far shore.

In the open expanses of water, you'll see dozens—if not hundreds—of birds, depending on the season. Sandhill cranes are common, obvious from their height. Spotting smaller wading birds, such as little blue herons, green herons, and white ibis, may take more time and some help from your zoom lens or binoculars. Redwing blackbirds appreciate the thickets of cattails; the birds' distinctive cries echo throughout the marsh. A series of small observation platforms and benches built into the boardwalk provides you plenty of perches for birding. But watch out for the scat, as it comes in many shapes, sizes, and consistencies, including splats.

The boardwalk jogs left and heads down another long straightaway, with the vast open spaces—prime feeding ground for wading birds—drawing closer on your right. After 1.2 miles the boardwalk ends at a platform with two benches, a good spot for watching raptors. Dog fennel grows thickly beyond this point, blocking your view. Backtrack along the boardwalk, taking your time to look for alligators, water snakes, and leopard frogs. By 1.6 miles you leave the boardwalk and climb back up the levee. Turn right and walk over to the observation deck, a roofed structure with a bench and a porch

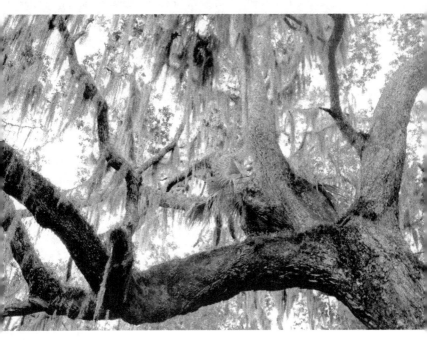

SAW PALMETTO GROWING IN THE CROOK OF A LIVE OAK TREE

swing overlooking the prairie. This is a great spot for additional birding in a patch of shade, as it looks over the open marsh.

Leaving the observation deck, walk back over the bridge to follow the footpath back the way you came. Although there is no marker alerting you to turn left, do so when you see the fence on the right, heading down the berm to your left to follow the grassy trail between the live oaks. After winding through the scrubby area and tracing your path back through patches of floodplain and pasture, you reach the forest road by 2.1 miles. Turn left. As the road curves to the right, stay with it, passing the main trail junction for a walk along the planted longleaf pine forest. Make a left at the double diamond markers to walk back to the parking area, completing your 2.5-mile hike.

Nearby Attractions

Grab breakfast or lunch at an iconic local restaurant, the Dam Diner, just south of the river along CR 464C. Hike 31, Carney Island Recreation & Conservation Area, is nearby. At the Silver River Museum (see Hike 37 or 38), you can see pre-Columbian stone heads—the only known examples in Florida—discovered here along the Ocklawaha River Basin.

Directions

From I-75, Exit 352, follow FL 40 east through Ocala and Silver Springs into the Ocala National Forest. After 19.3 miles turn south on CR 314A at the traffic light in Forest Corners. Follow this road south 6.6 miles, where it makes a sweeping left bend. Turn right onto SE 137th Avenue Road, which is next to a sign that says THE REFUGE AT OCKLAWAHA. Follow this limerock road for 0.8 mile to the preserve entrance on the left, marked by a small sign. The entry road is a little rough. Since this is a multiuse trail system, the parking area is especially large to accommodate horse trailers.

Rainbow Springs
State Park: Sandhill Nature Trail

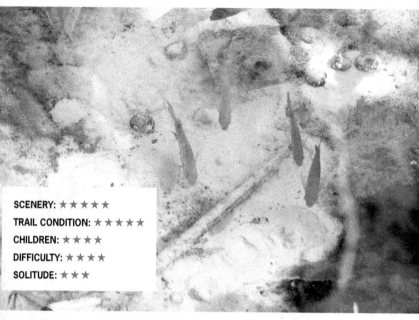

SCENERY: ★ ★ ★ ★ ★
TRAIL CONDITION: ★ ★ ★ ★ ★
CHILDREN: ★ ★ ★ ★
DIFFICULTY: ★ ★ ★ ★
SOLITUDE: ★ ★ ★

CRYSTALLINE WATERS AND TINY BUBBLING SPRINGS IN A RIVER COVE

GPS TRAILHEAD COORDINATES: N29° 06.250' W82° 26.316'

DISTANCE & CONFIGURATION: 4.4-mile balloon

HIKING TIME: 2 hours

HIGHLIGHTS: Spring and river views, fall wildflowers, historic phosphate pits

ACCESS: Daily, 8 a.m.–sunset. Entrance fee: $2 per person.

MAPS: USGS *Dunnellon*, at ranger station

FACILITIES: Concessions, gift shop, and restrooms near park entrance; picnic pavilions on far side of park; campground downriver accessed through separate entrance

WHEELCHAIR ACCESS: Limited to gardens; grades are steep.

COMMENTS: Leashed dogs welcome. The Sandhill Nature Trail begins a half mile from the parking area; full mileage, including the walk through the historic gardens, is included in the Route Details.

CONTACTS: Rainbow Springs State Park: 352-465-8555; **floridastateparks.org/rainbow springs.** Friends of Rainbow Springs State Park: 352-465-8555; **nccentral.com/FORS.**

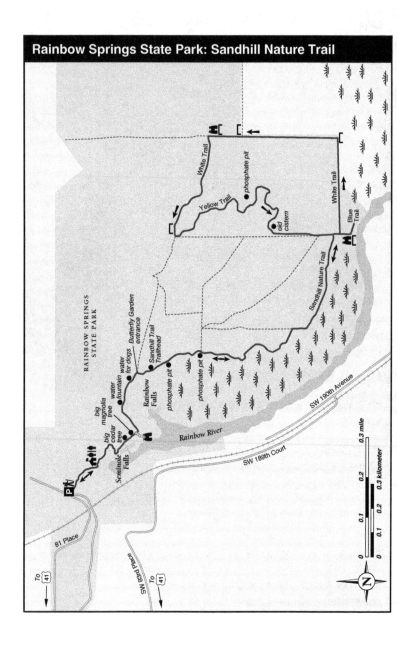

Rainbow Springs State Park: Sandhill Nature Trail

Overview

With steep bluffs overlooking the spring that produces one of the state's most beautiful rivers, the landscapes now protected by Rainbow Springs State Park have a long and storied history. It starts with the discovery of phosphate along the rivers around Dunnellon in 1890, creating a mining boom—and a town on this site, Juliette—by the turn of the 20th century. During the Great Depression, the hills were transformed into an attraction "to rival Silver Springs," with lush tropical plantings. Rainbow Springs, as it was called, remained a tourist attraction until the 1970s, when you could ride a leaf-shaped monorail through the gardens and aviary, look at the underwater splendor through the portholes of a submarine boat on a narrated cruise, or walk through zoo enclosures. Shuttered in 1973, it was at risk of becoming a subdivision. A county initiative raised the funds to buy the land, which was then turned over to Florida State Parks. After many years of loving restoration by volunteers, involving many residents who'd grown up with the attraction in their backyard, Rainbow Springs State Park fully opened in 1993.

Route Details

Showcasing the natural communities of the park, the Sandhill Nature Trail starts beyond the boundaries of the former attraction. To get there, the most direct route is a half-mile walk from the parking area, although you can take other side trips to lengthen that walk. Follow the broad sidewalk to the park's entrance, and pay your entrance fee. Ask for a trail map here. On the hillside overlooking the river and its springs, walk down the steps and take the path to the left, following its descent toward the river. Side trails lead uphill and toward a cove of crystalline water on a narrower path at the river's edge.

Past Seminole Falls, a boardwalk leads to a panorama of the river and another, larger cove. The main path sweeps past a shallow, clear pool filled with small, natural, bubbling springs before it turns past Rainbow Falls, the tallest of the man-made falls. As you climb uphill, follow the main path as it curves right toward the butterfly garden. You'll find a dog-watering station here and a water fountain near remnants of the old rodeo grounds and their stables. Take the first right when you enter the butterfly garden. The path crosses an old park road to the kiosk and the nature-trail sign that mark the trailhead of the Sandhill Nature Trail, a half-mile walk thus far.

Blazed with yellow, the trail is between two fences through an upland forest of laurel oaks. The fence discourages visitors from climbing down into the old mine pits, which, after a century, have filled in with the forest. At a fork in the trail, keep right, leaving the fence for a forest of oaks and pines. The landscape drops into more deep phosphate pits, filled with saw palmetto and tall trees, on the right. A split rail fence divides the trail from the steepest drop-offs. After so many decades of erosion and reforestation, these pits mimic natural ravines.

The trail continues straight ahead, where scrub understory plants coexist with laurel oaks, turkey oaks, and wiregrass. Tall slash pines stand along the edge of a pit to the right; a ribbon of saw palmetto runs through the understory. Keep right at the fork and follow the jog of the trail past older longleaf pines and the remnants of pines that have died due to infestation from Southern pine bark beetles. The canopy opens up as you emerge, after a mile, at a T intersection. Turn right to follow the blazes along this sand road/firebreak. Grasses and prickly pear cacti thrive beneath a cover of dog fennel in the open grassland.

At 1.2 miles you reach a trail junction where yellow blazes go left and blue blazes lead right. Turn right. You quickly come to the next junction. Continue straight ahead, following the blue blazes downhill. The trail leads you to a shady spot along the Rainbow River, where a bench invites you to sit and enjoy the scenery. Trail's end is at a small cove off the river; you can look out and see turquoise water, which signals one of the many small springs found along this river. A Florida Aquatic Preserve, the Rainbow River flows only 6 miles before emptying into the north-flowing waters of the Withlacoochee River on its way to the Gulf of Mexico.

Walk back along the river and up the hill to the trail junction, and turn right on the White Trail to start the loop portion of this hike. The trail is a broad path through pine flatwoods with a healthy understory of saw palmetto, transitioning to sandhills and scrub. At a bench, the trail reaches the property boundary of the park. Turn left and follow the barbed wire fence. Climbing uphill, you might notice a number of old bricks washing out of an eroded spot in the trail, perhaps remnants of the town of Juliette.

By 2 miles you reach the end of the fence. Beyond a bench and a sign with a white blaze pointing forward, the trail drops downhill and the landscape opens up dramatically into a healthy longleaf pine and wiregrass habitat. This section of the trail makes the walk up that fence line worthwhile. In the fall, you'll see blazing star, a tall, feathery bright purple wildflower, throughout this part of the forest. At the next trail junction, turn left to stay on the loop. As the forest becomes denser, shiny blueberry shows up along the trail. The path, still the width of a forest road, twists and winds through the oak hammock. Passing a white-tipped marker on the left that has "2B" carved into it, the trail reaches a junction of forest roads at a bench. A sign points forward, but the yellow-blazed trail—well worth taking—is to the left.

Turn left to follow the yellow blazes down a footpath into the laurel oak forest. Cabbage palms grow throughout this forest, and giant grapevines drape from the forest canopy. At 2.5 miles you climb up a mound, and soon after, find a split rail fence at a drop-off overlooking a very large phosphate pit, now a ravine filled with cabbage palms and very tall pines. The trail scrambles over and around mounds throughout this forest, all part of the phosphate diggings. You see a drop-off to the left near a log-shaped boulder. As you overlook the pit, you can clearly see a cliff face of solid limestone inside the diggings.

The trail turns right, away from the pit, and you see the sandhills to your left as the trail passes by a very old live oak with curving branches covered in resurrection fern. Crossing what looks like a dry waterway lined with cabbage palms, the trail parallels this dry streambed briefly before curving away from it toward a rainwater cistern.

Although no homes still exist from the mining town of Juliette that predated Rainbow Springs, this cistern was undoubtedly part of a homestead or mining complex during those busy years.

The yellow blazes lead you out of the forest and onto a sand road. Continuing down the hill, you quickly return to the start of the loop, the junction of the yellow and blue blazes, at 3.1 miles. Turn right to retrace the footpath toward its start. Keep alert for where the yellow blazes leave the edge of the prairie-topped hill and head back into the forest, beneath the tall pines and past the pits, to the nature trail's start at the kiosk.

Your hike on the Sandhill Nature Trail ends after 3.9 miles. Take your time walking back to the front entrance of the park, and explore the side paths along the way. Returning to your car, the minimum mileage you'll complete will be 4.4 miles.

Nearby Attractions

Rainbow River Canoe & Kayak rents watercraft and shuttles paddlers along this beautiful river run: **rainbowrivercanoeandkayak.com.** Summer brings tubing to the Rainbow River, with put-ins both at the state park campground and at KP Hole County Park, depending on the outfitter you use: **rainbowspringspark.com** or **kphole.com.** Bird's Underwater offers snorkeling and drift-dive trips on the river: **birds underwater.com.**

Directions

From I-75, Exit 352, follow FL 40 for 17.3 miles west to US 41. Turn south. The park entrance will be on the left after 0.7 mile. Follow the park road back to the main parking area. Rainbow Springs State Park is 3.8 miles north of downtown Dunnellon along US 41.

SCENERY: ★ ★ ★ ★
TRAIL CONDITION: ★ ★ ★ ★ ★
CHILDREN: ★ ★ ★ ★ ★
DIFFICULTY: ★
SOLITUDE: ★ ★

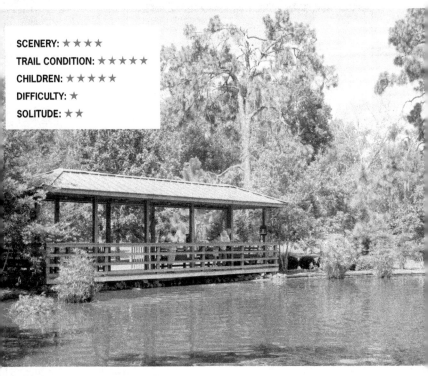

OBSERVATION DECK ON THE POND

GPS TRAILHEAD COORDINATES: N29° 06.896' W82° 15.360'

DISTANCE & CONFIGURATION: 1.6-mile double loop

HIKING TIME: 1 hour

HIGHLIGHTS: Labyrinth, gardens under ancient live oaks, the Pond

ACCESS: Daily, 8 a.m.–5 p.m. Daylight Saving Time: daily, 8 a.m.–7 p.m. Free.

MAPS: USGS *Dunnellon SE,* at trailhead kiosk

FACILITIES: Restrooms and water fountain, fish-feeding station at covered observation deck, benches all along trail system

WHEELCHAIR ACCESS: All trails are accessible except the Labyrinth.

COMMENTS: Dogs and bicycles are not permitted at Sholom Park, but the paved trails are perfect for wheelchairs and strollers. The fish food machine takes quarters.

CONTACTS: Sholom Park: 352-387-7404; **sholompark.com**

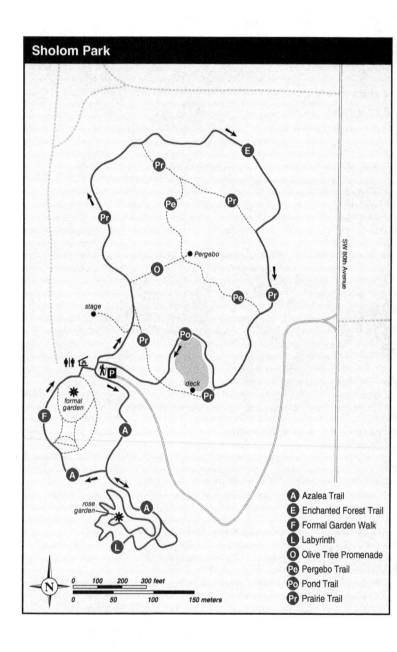

Sholom Park

SW 80th Avenue

Pergebo

stage

formal
garden

deck

rose
garden

N

0   100   200   300 feet

0   50   100   150 meters

A Azalea Trail
E Enchanted Forest Trail
F Formal Garden Walk
L Labyrinth
O Olive Tree Promenade
Pe Pergebo Trail
Po Pond Trail
Pr Prairie Trail

Overview

Walking as meditation: that's the goal at Sholom Park, a unique private nature park sculpted out of ranchland and remnants of hardwood hammock and climax sandhill forest. In the 1970s, Sidney Colen purchased Circle Square Ranch, nearly 13,000 acres of pasture and forest to the west of Ocala. He envisioned Sholom Park as a place for peaceful relaxation and reflection adjoining the expansive On Top of the World retirement community he built on the ranch. Opened in 2004, the park attracts all ages, young families and retirees, garden lovers and exercise walkers, with its blend of paved pathways, wild woodlands, and neatly groomed nature.

Route Details

There are many directions you can go and many paths you can take at Sholom Park; this hike is simply our recommended route through the 45-acre park. Start by walking up to the pavilion, where you can sign the guest register and pick up a map. You'll find restrooms and water fountains in this central location.

Turn left and face the fountain to enter the Formal Garden Walk, one of the most cultivated areas in the park, with changing beds of flowers and perennial foliage. Directly ahead are live oaks draped in Spanish moss, forming a frame for the garden view while deftly hiding the development beyond. You pass the first of many benches along the pathways of the park. Where a gravel path goes left, you come to a fork in the sidewalk. Keep right. The plantings throughout the park are a mixture of Florida natives and flora that require little to no watering. Hedges of azalea and boxwood form sculpted garden walls. There are many Southern magnolias, resplendent in aromatic blooms by late spring. The landscape dips to the left toward a sinkhole under the oaks. As the path curves to the edge of this formal area, follow it through a gate.

Walking beneath a very large hickory tree, you enter the Azalea Trail, where the blooms beneath these grand live oaks are at top form in February and early March. Walk past the junction of paths at a piece of statuary and continue straight ahead, downhill. You're on the outside of the Labyrinth looking in. It's one of the busier destinations in the park, particularly popular with children. Keep right at the fork in the trail, and enter the Labyrinth through a pergola covered in ivy. This is an out-and-back walk along a brick pathway. Many signs along the Labyrinth invite you to stop at various reflection points—such as the Wounded Heart Tree—and look at life from a different perspective. Longleaf pines tower over the neatly landscaped forest floor. Along this serpentine route, there are benches, arbors, gardens, and man-made water features beneath a canopy of live oaks laden with Spanish moss. At the heart of the Labyrinth, the brick path leads you around the Resting Tree, an immense hickory circled with benches, as it guides you back out the path you took to get here. Reaching the entrance pergola after 0.7 mile, turn right. Passing a bench, the trail loops back, rejoining the path that brought you to the Labyrinth. Continue straight ahead to the intersection with the statue. Turn right.

In the shade of the oaks among the azaleas, pass the next trail junction. A pathway comes in from the left, and you emerge at the parking area. Follow the path back past the pavilion. Just beyond the pavilion, turn left at the first break in the hedge and follow the path downhill into a vast, open setting on the Prairie Trail, where open grassy areas are edged with drought-resistant flower beds. Longleaf pines tower over the trails.

Past a side trail to a stage, you reach a triangular junction at 1 mile. To walk the perimeter of the park, keep left. Beyond a tablet with an inscribed poem, the Pergebo Trail—lined with olive trees—heads down to an open-air amphitheater used for weddings. Continue straight ahead. This part of the walk is in full sun, an easy place to notice the intentional impressions of leaves and fronds in the pathway.

As the pathway gains a little elevation, you can see the Enchanted Forest up ahead. It's a laurel oak forest, a climax sandhill, affording a return to shade. At the trail junction, turn left to enter the forest. Mistletoe grows profusely in the oaks' upper limbs. Squirrels dig through the leaf litter beneath the trees. A pileated woodpecker sounds like a doorknocker as it works its way through rotted wood.

The path curves right and leads you out of the forest, facing the big grassy area, coming to a T intersection with two benches at 1.3 mile. Turn left to rejoin the Prairie Trail. Stepping out into the sun, you're walking beneath big, beautiful longleaf pines. As the path draws much closer to the front gate, you hear traffic rushing by. Here, two big limestone boulders flank the trail, topped by homemade benches resplendent in mosses and ferns. The path curves right, meeting the other end of the Pergebo Trail. Surrounded by rocks is a poem about rocks. Continue straight ahead.

Although you're walking on a paved path, the forest floor around you is covered with pine duff. You hear the sound of water as you walk up toward the other child-attracting feature in this park, the Pond. Walk up to the Pond Deck and take a look over the side. The odd tint to the water keeps algae from growing and protects the fish

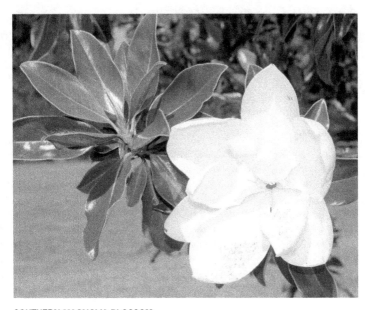

SOUTHERN MAGNOLIA BLOSSOM

from being easy pickings by osprey and herons. The koi are so used to being fed, they'll jump right out of the water for food. Turtles will paddle up, too, looking for their handouts.

Leaving the Pond Deck, take the time to walk around the pond itself to enjoy the panorama of the park from this elevated perspective. At the far end of the pond, water overflows on its own through a gravel bar when it gets too high. Passing the next bench on the right, continue straight ahead through the four-way intersection back to the parking area, completing the 1.6-mile hike.

Nearby Attractions

While the west side of Ocala is primarily residential, a short drive south on FL 200 leads you to the Ross Prairie Trailhead of the Cross Florida Greenway, with a campground, trails, and access to Ross Prairie State Forest: **floridahikes.com/hollyhammock.** You're also not far from Hike 28, Florida Trail: Southwest 49th Avenue to Land Bridge. Our favorite nearby restaurant is Crossroads Country Kitchen: **facebook.com/pages/Crossroads-Country-Kitchen/164746463581332.**

Directions

From I-75, Exit 350, follow FL 200 (SW College Road) southwest 3.9 miles through commercial and residential areas west of Ocala. Shortly after passing Queen of Peace Church, turn right on SW 80th Street and follow it 1.5 miles through a residential area. At the traffic light with SW 80th Avenue in front of Circle Square Commons, turn right and drive north. The park entrance is on the left after 0.7 mile. Follow the park road into Sholom Park, and choose from paved or grassy parking spaces.

Silver Springs
State Park: River Trails

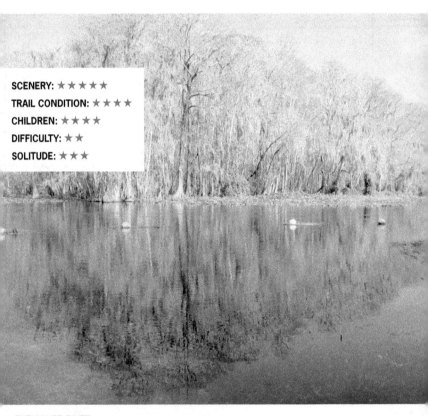

SCENERY: ★ ★ ★ ★ ★
TRAIL CONDITION: ★ ★ ★ ★
CHILDREN: ★ ★ ★ ★
DIFFICULTY: ★ ★
SOLITUDE: ★ ★ ★

THE SILVER RIVER

GPS TRAILHEAD COORDINATES: N29° 12.061' W82° 02.069'

DISTANCE & CONFIGURATION: 4.3-mile double balloon

HIKING TIME: 2 hours

HIGHLIGHTS: River views, birding, and interpretation

ACCESS: Daily, 8 a.m.–sunset. Entrance fee: $2 per pedestrian or cyclist; $4 per single-occupant vehicle; $8 for vehicle with up to 8 people.

MAPS: USGS *Ocala East*, at ranger station

Silver Springs State Park: River Trails

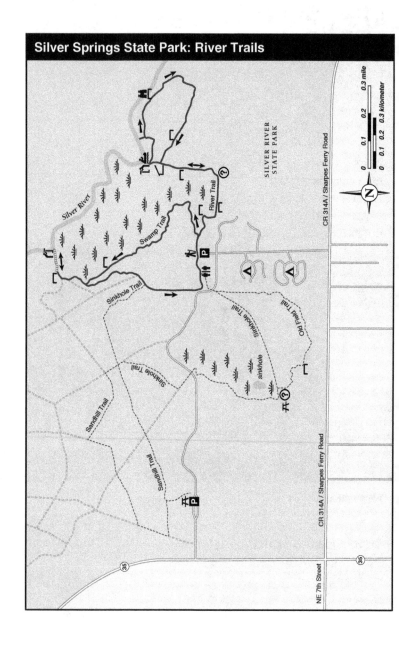

FACILITIES: Restrooms, picnic pavilions, playground, and campground near the trailhead; many benches along the trails. The Silver River Museum ($2 per person, under age 6 free) and Cracker Village are open only on weekends.

WHEELCHAIR ACCESS: None

COMMENTS: Leashed dogs welcome. Bicycles are permitted on this trail system but not on the boardwalks.

CONTACTS: Silver Springs State Park: 352-236-7148; **floridastateparks.org/silversprings.** Friends of Silver River State Park: **thefriendsofsilverriver.org.**

Overview

Renowned for its crystalline water and primordial beauty, the Silver River twists and winds through floodplain forests graced with ancient cypress, reaching the Ocklawaha River after a 6-mile journey. Its source is Silver Springs, one of the world's largest first-magnitude springs, pumping 550 million gallons of water a day out of the Floridan aquifer to the surface. Access to the springs is a new part of this state park. The River Trails offer a walk in the woods to several vantage points where you can enjoy the river flowing by. You can hike one or both of the trails. They also connect to the Sandhill and Sinkhole Trails (Hike 38), if you prefer to walk the full trail system in one go.

Route Details

Enter the River Trails through an archway from the parking area down a nice broad path. This trail system is made up of two popular trails, the Swamp Trail and the River Trail. At the junction of the two trails, keep right. The trail is a well-worn path through an upland hammock, winding beneath Southern magnolias and hickories. At the T intersection with the RIVER TRAIL sign, on the edge of the campground, turn left; follow the old road downhill. At the junction with the Ross Allen Trail, a mountain biking loop, the River Trail turns left to enter a floodplain forest. The old road provides just enough elevation to keep the trail out of the swamp. At 0.5 mile there is a bench in a clearing to the right of the trail. You emerge at a sunny spot with stacks of canoes. A kiosk and shaded bench—a tram stop at certain times of year—marks the beginning of the loop trail along the river. Before you head down it, take a walk down to the boardwalk and canoe-launch platform on the river's edge.

If you've never seen the crystalline waters of the Silver River, you'll be astounded at their clarity. Fish swim by as if suspended in air. Cormorants sit on logs on the far shore, drying their wings. The river indeed looks like a jungle, which is why it was used for the vine-swinging and underwater shots in Johnny Weissmuller's Tarzan movies in the 1930s and 1940s.

Leaving the canoe launch, walk along the edge of the forest to your left until you see a path paralleling the river. You walk past a cabbage palm resplendent in goldfoot fern and climbing aster. Looking left, you can see the line of cypress along the riverbanks. A side trail lets you creep right down to the river's edge between the cypress knees if the water is low. Watch carefully for alligators and cottonmouth moccasins. Back on the main trail, another side trail leads to a bench that looks out over the river at 1 mile. Another path to the left leads to the edge of the cypress floodplain amid towering trees with big knees. Past this point, the main trail turns away from the river to head back along the loop. Several fenceposts discourage you from taking an old side trail. The trail curves right to parallel a cypress strand. After passing a short cypress decorated in fungi and mosses, you come to another bench.

By 1.6 miles you return to the T intersection with the old road that led down to this area. Turn left to exit. When you reach the bike trail junction, turn right to walk up the hill out of the floodplain and into the upland forest. Turn right where you see the blue-tipped post at the corner by the cabins. Follow the meander of the River Trail back out to the main junction with the Swamp Trail, reaching it at 2.2 miles.

Turn right to continue your hike on the Swamp Trail. As the gentlest walk in the park, this is a favorite for families, and it starts under a large dahoon holly with a shape made for hugging. Resurrection fern covers the limbs of the live oaks throughout this forest. While this is primarily an upland hammock, there are little patches of scrub habitat throughout it. The Swamp Trail is marked with orange-tipped posts, and you'll find interpretive signs all along the trail, as well as mileage markers from the trailhead. As the trail winds through the forest, it stays in deep shade above the floodplain forest below.

Past a sabal palm interpretive sign, the trail curves left below the base of a very large live oak. Along this section, the live oaks dominate the forest, their trunks and limbs hosting hanging gardens of lichens and mosses. As the elevation changes, oaks take over, with saw palmetto thick in the understory. Watch for low-hanging oak limbs you must duck under. Where you see an old trail blocked off with logs, follow the Swamp marker straight ahead. Passing an abandoned side trail, the footpath flattens out near a collection of benches used for interpretive walks. In quick succession, two more trail markers guide you away from old trail routes, and you emerge at a T intersection with the tram road at 3 miles. Up ahead, the trail turns off the tram road and heads downhill to the floodplain.

Benches flank the entrance to the boardwalk that guides you through the floodplain forest of the Silver River. Crossing the cypress swamp, you may see tannic puddles between the trees and knees, or a sheet flow of water. The boardwalk ends at a dock and observation deck at the Silver River. Look into the water and notice the change in its color: you're above one of the many springs of the Silver River. It's easy to spend a long time staring down into the water, watching fish and turtles swim by. Resist the temptation to climb off the boardwalk, as there are always cottonmouth moccasins in the tree roots around this spot.

Backtrack along the boardwalk and up the hill to the tram road. Follow the markers up the tram road to the left to a footpath. Nicely shaded by the low canopy of the sand live oaks, the trail stays close to the ecotone. You pass several trail markers in quick succession. The purple hues of deer's-tongue and blazing star add color to this corridor in the fall. Old man's beard drapes thickly from the wizened oaks, looking like a seafoam-colored version of Spanish moss.

The trail winds through the oak scrub and continues to gain elevation. Crossing the tram road, you head into a sand pine scrub, coming to the junction with the Sinkhole Trail (Hike 38) at 3.7 miles. Continue straight ahead. The trails become a broad, long straightaway under a beautiful canopy of sand live oaks. At the end of the straightaway, the Swamp marker points you left. The trail narrows down and makes another jog left.

Turn left to walk along the edge of the playground and picnic complex. After a short stretch of scrub forest you emerge at a parking area. The restrooms are to your right. Turn left to continue up the last little piece of well-groomed trail past the Pioneer Village, emerging under the SINKHOLE TRAILS sign after 4.1 miles to the parking area, right across from the RIVER TRAILS sign.

Nearby Attractions

Don't miss Silver Springs itself. Ride the classic glass-bottomed boats, or paddle down the Silver River to see the many springs; walk the pathways through the riverside gardens. Adjacent Wild Waters provides summer splash time: **wildwaterspark.com.** Among its offerings, the Appleton Museum of Art showcases a significant collection of European art: **appletonmuseum.org.**

Directions

From I-75, Exit 352 (Ocala), follow FL 40 for 8.4 miles through Ocala to Silver Springs. Turn south on Baseline Road (FL 35), and continue another 1.1 miles to the park entrance on the left. Continue along the park road, passing the Sandhill Trailhead (Hike 38), and drive to the very end of the park to the large parking area adjacent to the Pioneer Village and Silver River Museum.

38 **Silver Springs State Park:** Sandhill and Sinkhole Trails

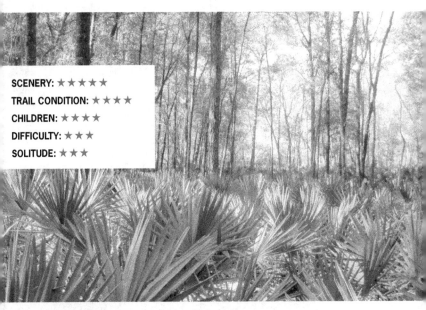

SCENERY: ★ ★ ★ ★ ★
TRAIL CONDITION: ★ ★ ★ ★
CHILDREN: ★ ★ ★ ★
DIFFICULTY: ★ ★ ★
SOLITUDE: ★ ★ ★

DENSE UNDERSTORY OF SAW PALMETTO ALONG THE SINKHOLE TRAIL

GPS TRAILHEAD COORDINATES: N29° 12.079' W82° 02.980'

DISTANCE & CONFIGURATION: 4-mile double loop

HIKING TIME: 2 hours

HIGHLIGHTS: Wildlife watching, interpretation, large live oaks

ACCESS: Daily, 8 a.m.–sunset. Entrance fee: $2 per pedestrian or cyclist; $4 per single-occupant vehicle; $8 for vehicle with up to 8 people.

MAPS: USGS *Ocala East,* at ranger station

FACILITIES: Picnic table at trailhead; restrooms, picnic pavilions, playground, and campground near the midpoint of the trail, where this trail connects with Hike 37; and the Silver River Museum ($2 per person, under age 6 free) and Cracker Village, open only on weekends

WHEELCHAIR ACCESS: None

COMMENTS: Leashed dogs welcome. Bicycles are permitted on this trail system. Be alert for wildlife encounters.

CONTACTS: Silver Springs State Park: 352-236-7148; **floridastateparks.org/silverriver.** Friends of Silver River State Park: **thefriendsofsilverriver.org.**

Silver Springs State Park: Sandhill and Sinkhole Trails

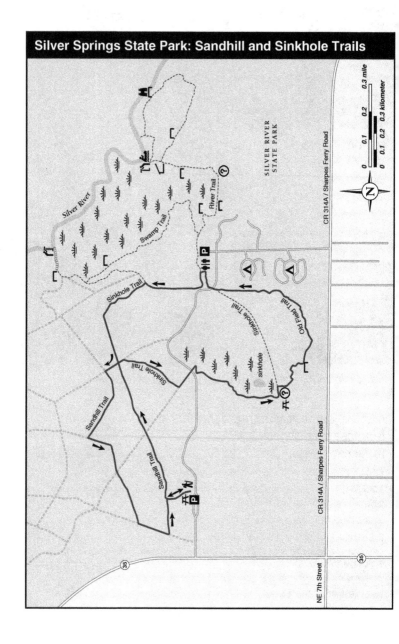

Overview

Since it opened in the 1980s, this state park protecting the south shore of the spring-fed Silver River had been known as Silver River State Park. In 2013, the park more than doubled in size when the former Silver Springs attraction, opened in the late 1800s, officially became part of the Florida State Parks system. The new name, Silver Springs State Park, encompasses it all. Just past the ranger station off Baseline Road, the Sandhill Trail is the easiest-to-access trailhead in the park, and one that never disappoints. It connects with the Sinkhole Trail, another major trail, which in turn connects to the River Trails (Hike 37). The Sandhill and Sinkhole Trails roam farther from the busy portions of the park, enough so that hikers sometimes see Florida black bears along them. The double loop creates a 4-mile hike.

Route Details

Step beneath the SANDHILL TRAIL sign, and start your walk into the sandhills. You step past a gopher tortoise burrow as longleaf pines loom tall overhead, sunlight filtering through their needles. Turn right at the T intersection to begin the loop. The sandhills are at their finest in fall, when wildflowers like blazing star, yellow buttons, golden aster, and Indian paintbrush lend their colors to nature's palette against a backdrop of wiregrass. You see the first trail marker, tipped in yellow, with an arrow and the word "Sandhill." Continue straight ahead.

Strewn with pinecones atop a soft layer of needles, the footpath is an inviting introduction to the trail system. Gopher apple, with its distinctive oval leaves, thrives in patches amid the wiregrass. You pass more trail markers, set at places where you might be tempted to follow an old side trail. The footpath becomes grassy, still a comfortable walk. Notice the shapes of the pine trees above? Several varieties grow here: loblolly, with its short, soft tufts of needles; slash pine, with longer needles; and longleaf pine, its needles a foot long or more. Their pinecones also provide a clue. The largest come from the longleaf. Sand pines, with very short, stiff needles, look the most like Christmas trees and have hard nuggetlike cones.

Passing interpretive markers for wiregrass and wild plum, you can see a change in the habitat as the trail starts a gentle climb. There are now prominent clumps of saw palmetto in the understory, and the pines and turkey oaks are shorter. At 0.7 mile you reach a well-marked intersection for the Sandhill and Sinkhole Trails at a kiosk and picnic bench. You'll return to this point later in the hike; turn right to start this loop. Past a tall cluster of saw palmetto, you reach a SINKHOLE trail sign. Turn right, passing a cabbage palm. The forest crowds in on both sides, but the trail is still very broad. Past an oak thickly laden with Spanish moss, make a sharp left at a T intersection. You cross the park road at 1.1 miles.

The trail continues past a split rail fence downhill into a more mature forest, facing the park road briefly before making a sharp left deeper into the shade. Clumps of saw palmetto dominate the understory. Past a Sinkhole marker, notice how the landscape drops off dramatically into the sinkhole. It's most noticeable in winter when the deciduous trees lose their leaves. The interior of the sinkhole is wooded and marshy, dense with willows. The trail veers right, away from the sinkhole itself, to meet a T intersection with a service road. Turn left. You walk up to a kiosk with a trail map, a couple of picnic benches, and the junction with the Old Field Loop at 1.5 miles. Turn right.

The Old Field Loop is just what it says—a loop through an old field, which, after nearly 30 years of forest growth, is looking pretty nice as the sandhill and scrub naturally reclaim the land. There are many interpretive signs along this trail. Winding through the forest, the trail is not an obvious footpath, but yellow-tipped markers point the way. As the trail enters deeper shade, the live oaks around you are distinctly beautiful, massive trees with long limbs covered in a thick blanket of mosses, lichens, and resurrection fern. An oak and pine have grown together, forming a crooked "H" at their bases.

The trail reaches the campground at 2.1 miles. Turn left. You follow the edge of the campground along a broad path before merging back into the Sinkhole Trail to cross the park road. Walk straight ahead, paralleling the edge of the park road by a picnic area and playground, to meet the junction with the Swamp Trail. The Swamp Trail is part of Hike 37, starting at a trailhead that's up the path to the right. That side trail also leads to the "populated" part of the park, if you wish to visit the restrooms and water fountain, or the Cracker Village and Silver River Museum (open on weekends). Otherwise, continue straight ahead.

Shaded by rusty lyonia, the Sinkhole Trail parallels the park road up to where the orange marker says SWAMP and the red marker says SINKHOLE. Turn right to walk down a nicely shaded corridor through the scrub forest. As the straightaway curves, turn left at the SINKHOLE TRAIL sign. Losing elevation, the footpath is now bright white sand beneath the sand live oaks. The corridor opens up into bright sun with patches of blueberries. You reach a T intersection; turn left. As you walk through sandy spots, look down and you'll see tracks from deer, raccoons, and sometimes even bobcats or bears.

By 3 miles you return to the original junction of the Sinkhole and Sandhill Trails at the kiosk and picnic bench. It's now time to complete the Sandhill Trail loop. Turn right. At a four-way intersection, two directions are marked with SERVICE ROAD signs, and you came from the third direction, so turn left, following the SANDHILL sign. This part of the trail is broad like an old forest road, but you're firmly back in a sandhill forest again. An undulation to the left might be a sinkhole; across from it, the trail turns right onto a narrower path. The straightaway is broken only by a single oak with a cluster of saw palmetto beneath it.

At the next T intersection, the trail turns left at 3.5 miles, leading you deeper into a robust sandhill forest. Fire management is a necessary part of tending to sandhill habitat, which is why you'll see burn marks up the trees and, occasionally, firebreaks churning up part of this trail, making hiking challenging. Where you see the next sign for a service road, the trail turns right, onto a grassy footpath surrounded by younger pines. Keep alert at the next trail marker and you'll spot a gopher tortoise burrow nearby. When you reach a forest road with a sign pointing left, you can hear traffic from nearby Baseline Road. Scattered bracken fern emerges from the thick matting of wiregrass and oak leaves on the forest floor.

Just as you start to see some utility wires to the right, the trail turns away from the park perimeter and makes a sharp left. The turkey oak forest sweeps down from both sides toward the footpath. In winter, you can see the roof of the ranger station to the right as you approach the end of the loop. At the signs for the parking lot and ranger station, turn right to exit, emerging at the parking area after 4 miles.

Nearby Attractions

Generations have delighted in a cruise down the Silver River in a glass-bottomed boat; make sure you have your turn during a visit to this delightful park. Canoe and kayak rentals are available, along with mountain biking trails and campsites and cabins in a shady forested setting. On weekends, the Silver River Museum is well worth a visit; the Cracker Village is at its best during Ocali Country Days, held each November: **marion.k12.fl.us/district/srm/ocali.cfm.**

Directions

From I-75, Exit 352 (Ocala), follow FL 40 for 8.4 miles through Ocala to Silver Springs. Turn south on Baseline Road (FL 35), and continue another 1.1 miles to the park entrance on the left. Outlined by a split rail fence, the trailhead is immediately on the left after the ranger station.

Appendix A: Outdoor Retailers

While many outlets—from drugstores to supercenters—carry items that would be useful on the trail, the following retailers carry hiking gear. The oldest outfitter in the region, Brasingtons Adventure Outfitters, draws hikers from around the region because of its very specific hiking and backpacking focus.

BRASINGTONS ADVENTURE OUTFITTERS
2331 NW 13th St.
Gainesville, FL 32609
352-372-0521
888-438-4502
brasingtons.com

BUCK N' BASS
14100 North FL 19
Salt Springs, FL 32134
352-685-0200
bucknbasssports.com

FLINT CREEK OUTFITTERS
4414 SW College Rd., #910
Ocala, FL 34474
352-237-5325
flintcreekoutfitters.com

GANDER MOUNTAIN
3970 SW Third St., #101
Ocala, FL 34474
352-351-6186
gandermountain.com

 # Appendix B: Map Resources

Visitor centers and ranger stations generally provide free maps of the trails. For maps of the Florida Trail, you can order online or stop at the Florida Trail Association office on US 441 in Gainesville, which is open Monday–Friday, 9 a.m.–4 p.m. It also carries T-shirts, books, and some hiking gear.

FLORIDA TRAIL ASSOCIATION
5415 SW 13th St.
Gainesville, FL 32608
352-378-8823
floridatrail.org

Stop in at the National Forest visitor centers on FL 40 near Silver Springs or FL 19 at Salt Springs for maps. You can also download maps for non–Florida Trail hikes in the Ocala National Forest from the Ocala National Forest website under the Maps and Publications link: **fs.usda.gov/ocala.**

Maps for hikes on St. Johns Water Management District lands are available both in their free *Recreation Guide to District Lands* and on their website: **sjrwmd.com /recreationguide.**

The City of Gainesville Parks and Recreation Department, Nature Operations Division, plans to provide printable park maps on their website: **natureoperations.org.**

Download GPS tracks of the trails in this book: **floridahikes.com/fivestargainesvilleocala.**

Appendix C: Hiking Clubs

The clubs listed below have long, stable histories and welcome visitors to their meetings. All clubs welcome nonmembers to their meetings and to some of their activities.

FLORIDA TRAIL ASSOCIATION, FLORIDA CRACKERS CHAPTER
5415 SW 13th St.
Gainesville, FL 32608
floridatrail.orgmeetup.com/crackers-fta
Annual dues: $30–$35 (for statewide membership) *Check the website for meeting times and locations, which vary.*

FLORIDA TRAIL ASSOCIATION
Halifax–St. Johns Chapter
Palatka, FL, and Deland, FL
floridatrail.org
Annual dues: $30–$35 (for statewide membership) *See Florida Trail Association website for meeting times and locations.*

SUWANNEE–ST. JOHN'S SIERRA CLUB
P.O. Box 13951
Gainesville, FL 32604
ssjsierra.org
Annual dues: $39 (for nationwide membership) *Meetings are held on the first Thursday of each month 7 p.m.–9:30 p.m. at the Unitarian Universalist Fellowship of Gainesville.*

You'll find additional gatherings of Gainesville and Ocala–area hikers on Meetup **meetup.com**, including the popular North Florida Explorers, **meetup.com/hiking-270.**

Index

Check out this other great title from
—— Menasha Ridge Press! ——

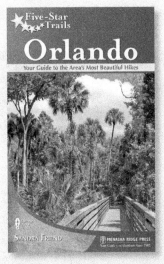

Five-Star Trails Orlando

by Sandra Friend   5x8, paperback
ISBN: 978-0-89732-922-7   264 pages
$15.95   maps, photographs, and index

Orlando is Florida's epicenter of spectacular hiking trails and
your launch pad to outdoor adventure. Covering 37 hikes across
a compact five-county region, all within an hour's drive of downtown Orlando and the theme parks, *Five-Star Trails Orlando*
gives you a reason to get outdoors now! Authored by Florida
hiking expert and local resident Sandra Friend, this handy guide
offers a mix of gentle, family-friendly nature trails, easy day
hikes, and more strenuous immersions through vast wild spaces.
Friend's vivid hike descriptions give insight to the history, flora,
and fauna of the routes, and her concise, accurate trail directions
and mileages will keep explorers on the right path.

MENASHA RIDGE PRESS
www.menasharidge.com
Your Guide to the Outdoors Since 1982

AR CUSTOMERS AND FRIENDS,

PORTING YOUR INTEREST IN OUTDOOR ADVENTURE, travel, and an
ive lifestyle is central to our operations, from the authors we choose to
 locations we detail to the way we design our books. Menasha Ridge
ss was incorporated in 1982 by a group of veteran outdoorsmen and
fessional outfitters. For many years now, we've specialized in creating
oks that benefit the outdoors enthusiast.

host immediately, Menasha Ridge Press earned a reputation for
olutionizing outdoors- and travel-guidebook publishing. For such
ivities as canoeing, kayaking, hiking, backpacking, and mountain
ing, we established new standards of quality that transformed the
ole genre, resulting in outdoor-recreation guides of great sophisti-
ion and solid content. Menasha Ridge continues to be outdoor
blishing's greatest innovator.

e folks at Menasha Ridge Press are as at home on a white-water river or
untain trail as they are editing a manuscript. The books we build for you
 the best they can be, because we're responding to your needs. Plus, we
e and depend on them ourselves.

 look forward to seeing you on the river or the trail. If you'd like to
ntact us directly, join in at www.trekalong.com or visit us at
w.menasharidge.com. We thank you for your interest in our books
d the natural world around us all.

FE TRAVELS,

Bob Sehlinger

B SEHLINGER
BLISHER

About the Authors

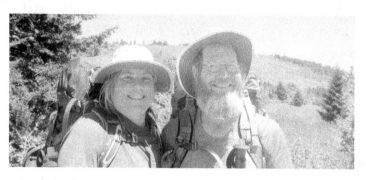

A hiker since she was old enough to toddle through the Appalachians with her parents, **SANDRA FRIEND** is known as Florida's hiking expert, having logged more than 3,500 miles on foot throughout the state. Known best for her nature writing, Sandra is also a travel writer. A member of the Society of American Travel Writers and the Florida Outdoor Writers Association, she has authored or coauthored 28 books since 1999, more than half of them about her home state of Florida; written three smartphone apps; and collaborated on an active travel website, **buckettripper.com.** An avid photographer, Sandra enjoys sharing her outdoor experiences around the world.

A native Floridian growing up along the Space Coast, **JOHN KEATLEY** spent most of his youth in the woods or on the water with the Boy Scouts, becoming an Eagle Scout. During a 33-year career on the Space Shuttle program, he found time between missions to unwind in the great outdoors, camping, sailing, canoeing, hiking, and cycling. As the shuttle program came to an end, he resumed the outdoor activities he loved as a youth and began a new career as an outdoor writer. While preparing for a thru-hike of the Appalachian Trail, he met Sandra, and they have been hiking and writing together ever since. John is a member of the Florida Outdoor Writers Association and enjoys sharing his unique stories of outdoor adventure.

Follow Sandra and John's adventures at **floridahikes.com** and **trails andtravel.com.**

Printed in the USA
CPSIA information can be obtained
at www.ICGtesting.com
JSHW011521130424
61126JS00002B/5